The Longevity
BLUEPRINT

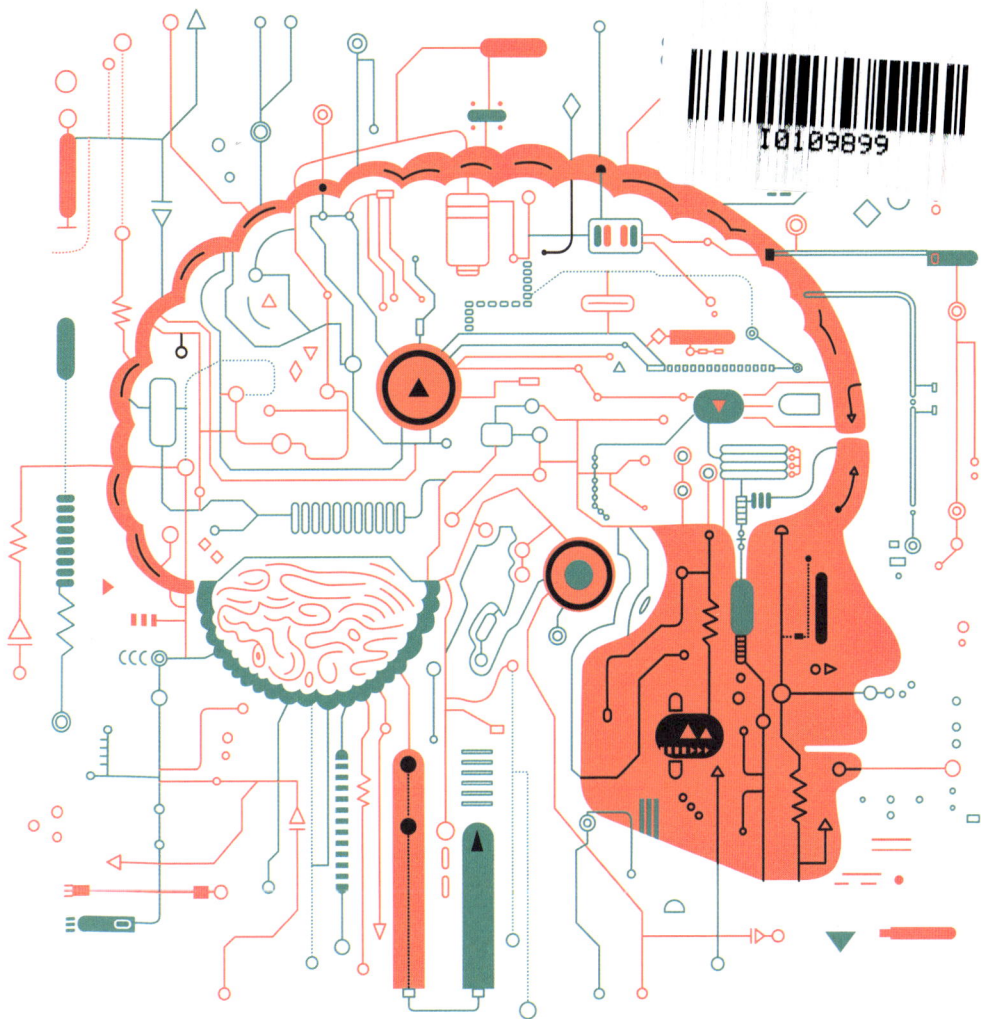

chartwell
books

Contents

Introduction

"Everyone Desires Long Life, Not One Old Age."

Jonathan Swift

Medical and technological advances and interventions today have enabled us to live longer and live better. But along with longevity, there's an increasing prevalence in certain degenerative diseases such as Alzheimer's disease and other forms of dementia; cardiovascular diseases, diabetes, and certain types of cancer. What if you could reverse-engineer your body and mind to improve your health and well-being? What if you could not only prolong your life but prolong your quality of life by making simple modifications to your lifestyle?

Drawn from fields including biology, genetics, neuroscience and nutrition, biohacking describes the practice of enhancing physical or mental performance to improve well-being or to achieve specific health outcomes. To 'biohack your brain,' or to 'DIY your biology,' may sound like something out of science fiction. If you've heard of biohacking, you might associate it with expensive techniques and technology such as EEG (electroencephalogram) devices or transcranial magnetic stimulation to optimize cognitive function and mental well-being. Those are indeed methods of heightening your brain's performance and resilience. However, you can also achieve results through targeted, incremental interventions that are based on science and personal lifestyle experimentation to discover what works for you. In other words, there are many hacks that you can do for free.

Simple but powerful habits, such as nourishing your body with nutrient-dense foods, prioritizing restorative sleep, and practicing mindfulness, can profoundly impact brain and bodily function. Balanced nutrition supplies the building blocks for neurotransmitters, while consistent, high-quality sleep consolidates memory, enhances learning, and supports emotional regulation. Mindfulness training lowers stress hormones, improves focus, and fosters resilience, creating an optimal mental environment for neuroplastic change.

Neuroplasticity — the brain's ability to rewire itself—allows the body's 'supercomputer' to change and adapt throughout life. The brain forms new connections, reorganizes existing ones, and even creates new neurons in response to learning, experience, or injury. Essentially, your brain is constantly rewiring itself based on what you do, think, and feel. Learning a new skill or habit, for example, allows your brain to form new neural pathways to support that activity.

Through small, strategic changes to your lifestyle, environment, and biology, you can enhance your mental performance, health, and well-being, improving your quality of life in the long term. In this book, we'll explore lifestyle changes that can help you to sharpen your mind, unlock your brain's full capacity, and protect it against the cognitive decline that comes with age. You'll learn more about the role of nutrition, exercise, sleep, mental stimulation, and mindfulness in profoundly shaping your brain's function.

Your brain and body are capable of remarkable change. It's never too late to enhance your physical and mental well being and with the right strategies, you'll begin to see improvements. Whether you're looking to be more productive, more creative, or simply maintain sharp cognitive function well into old age, this book is your blueprint to becoming the best version of yourself, mentally and cognitively. Are you ready? Let's get started.

Nutrition

A

Nutrition

Making changes to your daily diet can help to optimize your cognitive function, mental clarity, mood, and overall brain health. Proper nutrition is a great first step for providing your brain and body with the right building blocks and energy sources to keep them running a peak performance. Here's a little background on the brain-nutrition connection. While these two subjects may seem unrelated, they are inextricably linked.

The foods you eat and the liquids you drink contain stored chemical energy that your body breaks down into smaller components so it can absorb them to use as fuel. Energy comes from the three main nutrients: carbohydrates, protein, and fats, with carbohydrates (glucose, for example) being the most important source. In cases where carbohydrates have been depleted, your body can use protein and fats for energy.

To understand how energy is used in your brain and body, you need to understand the metabolism. That's the word that describes the chemical reactions taking place in the body's cells that convert food into energy. An optimal metabolism requires sufficient nutrients received from the consumption of foods and liquids. If you don't get them, the metabolism underperforms, and you feel tired and sluggish.

All foods provide you with energy. But some foods are more efficient at boosting energy levels, such as bananas (an excellent source of carbohydrates, potassium and vitamin B6), fatty fish such as salmon or tuna (good sources of protein, fatty acids and B vitamins), brown rice (a source of fiber, vitamins and minerals), and eggs (source of protein). Foods packed with carbohydrates, fiber, or protein slowly release energy and essential vitamins, minerals, and antioxidants so they can be sustained over a longer period of time.

The rate at which the body uses food energy to sustain life and to do different activities is called the metabolic rate. The total energy conversion rate when we are at rest is called the *basal metabolic rate* (BMR) and is divided among various systems in your body, with the largest part going to the liver and spleen, followed by the brain. The BMR is a function of age, gender, total body weight, and amount of muscle mass (which burns more calories than body fat). About 75 percent of food calories are used to sustain basic body functions included in the basal metabolic rate.

If you need more energy than you consume, such as when you're doing vigorous work, your body draws upon the chemical energy stored in your body fat, which is why exercise can be helpful in losing fat. However, the amount of exercise needed to produce a loss in fat, or to burn off extra calories consumed that day, can be a lot. The most important thing to remember with physical energy is that you have the power to make food and drink choices that can significantly improve how your body functions, metabolizes food, and both stores and utilizes energy. That means you can improve how your body and brain function.

Though it's typically about 2 percent of your body weight, your brain consumes 20 to 25 percent of your metabolic energy—and that's when it's keeping your 86 billion neurons and give-or-take 164 trillion synapses on stand-by. Once activated, your brain's energy needs skyrocket. It requires significant energy to suppress distractions, pay attention, process information, analyze situations, find solutions, think creatively, make decisions, conduct conversations, access memory, maintain self-control, feel and express empathy, or even meditate.

Even when you aren't aware that your brain is working—while mindlessly perusing TV channels to find entertainment, laughing, or daydreaming, for example—it is tapping into whatever mental energy you've accrued. Your brain is quite literally at the heart of everything you do and sets the agenda for doing anything at all.

To do the tasks it's asked to do, your brain needs oxygen, glucose, and a full suite of macro- and micronutrients. When its energy levels aren't sufficient, your brain will usurp your physical energy. Needing more oxygen, it can send messages to your heart to pump faster, which can lead to increased blood pressure.

Monitor Your Food-Energy Connection

Paying attention to your energy levels can help you to make a connection between what you eat and how you feel. Depending on what you eat, you may experience physical weakness or fatigue or mental fatigue, manifesting as difficulty concentrating, mood changes (such as irritability or anxiety), low motivation, or slower thinking and processing. Keeping a journal can you help identify patterns, and make you more aware of subtle shifts throughout the day. Persistent low energy may not just be about your nutritional habits: it may point to underlying medical issues such as anemia, thyroid disorders, or chronic fatigue syndrome. Increasing your awareness of the links between your food and energy levels will help you determine if what you're experiencing is diet related or something else.

By consistently monitoring these signs and reflecting on your experiences, you can better understand your energy patterns, identify what boosts or drains you, and take steps to improve it.

What changes in your energy do you notice within two hours after eating?

_____

_____

_____

_____

_____

_____

_____

Which foods tend to leave you feeling energized, and which make you feel sluggish?

_____

_____

_____

_____

_____

_____

_____

_____

_____

_____

"I don't think I'll ever grow old and say, 'What was I thinking eating all those fruits and vegetables?'"

Nancy S. Mure

How does skipping a meal affect your concentration and mood?

_____

_____

_____

_____

_____

_____

_____

_____

After eating a large meal, what happens to your activity level and alertness?

_____

_____

_____

_____

_____

_____

_____

_____

_____

How does your hydration level influence your daily energy patterns?

_____

_____

_____

_____

_____

_____

_____

_____

_____

What can you identify as nutritional changes you'd need to make to improve your brain's energy supply?

_____

_____

_____

_____

_____

_____

_____

_____

_____

_____

What does a typical day of eating look like for you? Describe meals, snacks, and drinks from morning to night.

_____

_____

_____

_____

_____

_____

_____

_____

What types of foods do you crave most often? What might those cravings be telling you?

_____

_____

_____

_____

_____

_____

_____

_____

_____

_____

What role does convenience play in your food choices?

_____

_____

_____

_____

_____

_____

_____

_____

_____

Which nutrition factors can you identify as depleting the energy that's getting to your brain?

_____

_____

_____

_____

_____

_____

_____

_____

_____

_____

Diet Dangers

The food and drink choices you make will affect your mental energy. Some of the common nutrition pitfalls that affect your brain performance include these stumbling blocks.

Eating Too Much Sugar

Sugary foods spike your blood sugar increasing your energy and alertness temporarily, but soon lead to a crash, resulting in a fatigue and irritability. While sweets may be the obvious problem, refined carbohydrates (white bread, crackers, chips, cereal) are also a major source of sugar. Balance your meals with fiber-rich carbohydrates, lean protein, and healthy fats.

Skipping Breakfast

After fasting while asleep, your body needs fuel. Skipping breakfast denies your body the fuel it needs and makes you more likely to make poor food choices later. Combining healthy carbohydrates (fruit, veggies, whole grains) with a protein source (eggs, nuts, dairy) gives you an initial boost and helps you make a healthy choice for lunch.

Consuming Too Much Caffeine

Caffeine provides a quick jolt but can also lead to crashes that leave you feeling fatigued, irritable, and unable to concentrate. It can also affect how well you sleep, so limit it to no more than four six-ounce servings a day, and switch to water or herbal tea in the afternoon.

Dehydration

Even mild dehydration can affect your energy level, mood, and ability to concentrate. Try to drink at least one glass of water per hour and be sure to fill your bottle up even more if you're exercising or are outdoors in high temperatures.

Poor Snacking Choices

Snacking on ultra-processed carbs depletes your energy. If you're going to snack (and it's good to snack), choose foods that provide protein and fiber, such as cheese, fruit, whole-grain toast with almond butter, or a few slices of chicken or turkey and baby carrots.

Excessive Eating

When you eat a big meal, it diverts blood to your digestion system, depriving your brain of oxygen and making you feel sluggish. Instead, choose portion-controlled, balanced meals that feature lean protein, complex carbohydrates (starchy vegetables, whole grains, beans, lentils), healthy fats, and lots of vegetables.

"Don't eat anything your great grandmother wouldn't recognize as food. When you pick up that box of portable yogurt tubes, or eat something with 15 ingredients you can't pronounce, ask yourself, "What are those things doing there?"

Michael Pollan,
In Defense of Food: An Eater's Manifesto

Food for Thought

Choosing foods with the most bang for their buck health-wise can make an immediate difference in creating, sustaining, and boosting your energy levels. Obviously, making lifestyle changes, and sustaining them over time, will improve your ability to create, maintain, and boost energy levels. Let's discuss specifics!

Eat More Complex Carbs

When your blood sugar dips too low or spikes too high, your energy levels are imbalanced, causing hunger, irritability, and difficulty concentrating. Complex carbohydrates should be a regular part of your diet. To maintain a healthy balance, choose the following:

◊   **Whole grains.** A good source of fiber, potassium, magnesium, and selenium

◊   **Fiber-rich fruits.** Apples, berries, and bananas, for example. Berries typically contain antioxidants and blueberries help with optimal brain performance. When necessary, frozen fruit is a great alternative to fresh, as the nutrients are typically sealed in during the freezing process. Avoid canned fruit since it usually contains added syrup.

◊   **Fiber-rich vegetables.** All vegetables contain complex carbohydrates and fiber. Especially strong choices are broccoli, leafy greens, and carrots. Toss spinach or kale into smoothies for a green boost.

◊   **Beans.** Aside from fiber, beans are good sources of folate, iron, and potassium.

◊   **Nuts and seeds.** Many contain good fats (see below), but most are also fattening, so eat them in moderation.

Which of the foods mentioned on page 18 are missing from your daily diet?

_____

_____

_____

_____

_____

_____

If you are not eating energy-enhancing food, what's stopping you from doing so? What would it take to make you eat more of them? What steps could you take to make that happen?

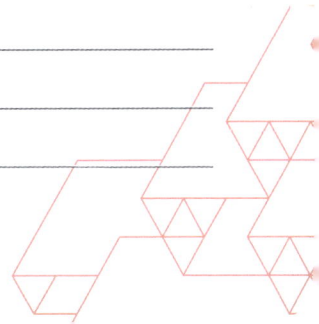

_____

_____

_____

_____

_____

_____

_____

_____

_____

Eat Seasonal Fruits and Vegetables

Unlike processed foods that may be stripped of nutrients for a longer shelf life, fresh foods are higher in nutrients. Eating in-season fruits and vegetables means they ripened naturally and will offer you the most bang for your energy buck.

Best Veggies

The best vegetables to eat according to nutritionist Dave Asprey's *Bulletproof Diet* are:

◊ Organic, when possible

◊ Best: asparagus, avocado (raw), bok choy, broccoli, brussels sprouts, cauliflower, celery, cucumber, fennel, olives.

◊ Next best: cabbage, collard greens, kale, lettuce, radishes, spinach, summer squash, zucchini.

Dave Asprey, The Bulletproof Diet: Lose Up to a Pound a Day, Reclaim Energy and Focus, Upgrade Your Life (Emmaus, PA: Rodale Books, 2014).

Top Ten Fiber-Rich Fruits

Raspberry	Papaya	Fig
Blackberry	Orange	Avocado
Strawberry	Apple	
Prune	Pear	

Go Bananas

When the National Institutes of Health asked long-distance cyclists to replace carbohydrate sports drinks with bananas, they found that bananas offered just as much fuel to the riders as the drinks. Bananas are filled with potassium, fiber, vitamins, and the perfect amount of carbohydrates to provide a big boost of natural energy. Plus, they're affordable!

"Eat good food, not too much, mostly plants."

Michael Pollan
author of *In Defense of Food*

Reduce Ultra-Processed Foods

One of the most important ways to maintain high energy levels is to avoid eating highly processed foods, such as some packaged or canned foods, candy, cookies and other packaged sweets, boxed meals, and precooked meats. These are typically high in added sugar, salt, unhealthy fats, and chemical additives, preservatives, sodium, trans fat, and artificial ingredients that may slow you down. Packaged foods are typically very easy to digest, which can lead to big blood sugar peaks followed by dips. According to food guru Michael Pollan, you should avoid the center aisles in grocery stores, avoid anything with more than five ingredients, or ingredients you can't pronounce, and, with the exception of honey, don't eat anything that doesn't rot.

Which ultra-processed foods do you need to eliminate or at least dramatically pare back?

Reflect upon your relationship with these foods. What makes them appealing to you--the taste, convenience, or emotional connection? Knowing they are not good for you, what makes them hard to give up?

Action Note

Use the space below to create a list of all the additives you want to avoid. Use this when grocery shopping to eliminate foods that drain rather than boost energy.

_____

_____

_____

_____

_____

_____

Ultra-Processed Foods to Avoid

Sugary and Sweetened Products
Candy, chocolate bars, and sweet snacks
Sugary breakfast cereals
Packaged pastries, cookies, and cakes
Ice cream and frozen desserts with additives

Sweetened and Artificial Beverages
Soda and energy drinks
Flavored or sweetened coffee/tea drinks
Fruit drinks (not 100% juice)
Sports drinks

Processed Snacks and Convenience Foods
Chips, cheese puffs, and similar snacks
Instant noodles and flavored pasta/rice packets
Frozen pizzas and microwave meals
Ready-to-eat packaged sandwiches/burgers

Processed Meats
Hot dogs, sausages, and deli meats
Bacon
Breaded chicken nuggets or patties
Meat sticks or jerky with additives

Dairy and Dairy-like Products
Flavored yogurt with added sugars
Cheese spreads and processed cheese slices
Non-dairy creamers with hydrogenated oils

Other Highly Processed Items
Margarine and shortening with trans fats
Flavored instant soups
Condiments with added sugars
Meal replacement shakes

Eat More Super Grains

Super grains are foods that provide high nutritional value with minimal fat or sugar. They typically digest slowly, which helps prevent blood sugar levels from spiking or dipping, both of which negatively impact your energy. Many of these super grains also benefit your gut bacteria. Some grains you can easily add to your diet include the following.

Oats: Helpful in reducing the risk of colon cancer and lower blood pressure, they also lower "bad" LDL cholesterol and total cholesterol.

Whole Grain Bread: Look for bread high in fiber with visible grains or seeds.

Whole Grain Rye: High in dietary fiber, this grain can slow down the absorption of carbs to create a slow but steady rise in blood sugar.

Buckwheat: Full of nutrients such as manganese, magnesium, copper, phosphorus, iron, B vitamins and fiber, this is a gluten-free grain.

Quinoa: Contains all nine essential amino acids.

Pop Your Own Popcorn

Popcorn is a whole-grain food high in important nutrients like manganese, magnesium, zinc, copper, phosphorus and many B vitamins. It's also incredibly high in fiber—3.5 ounces (100 grams) provide 14.5 grams of fiber or 58 percent of daily requirements. Steer clear of prepacked popcorn as it has chemicals; pop your own, just don't saturate it with butter.

Eat Often and Light

A good way to keep up your energy through the day is to eat regular meals and healthy snacks every three to four hours, rather than a large meal less often. It's also good to stop eating before you're full, which will help your body digest the food.

On the Whole

Studies show that people who eat the most whole grains live the longest and have the best health and least disease. Rice is the most consumed food on earth, followed closely by wheat. Millet, oats, barley, corn, buckwheat, and rye are eaten less, but offer many health benefits, too.

Whole grains have not been processed, cracked, or broken. When a grain is ground, oxidation starts and the oil in the grain can become rancid over time. Processing removes both the bran and germ of the grain—its most nutrient-rich component. Processing also removes more than half of vitamins B1, B2, B3, and E, as well as folic acid, calcium, phosphorus, zinc, copper, iron, and fiber. Once grain is cracked or ground into flour, it contains less vitality for daily food.

Whole grains contain all the major nutrient groups—complex carbohydrates, amino acids, protein, fats, vitamins, minerals, and fiber. The B-complex vitamins support a strong immune system. Whole grains help sustain your blood sugar levels and balance hormones. They provide antioxidants and regulate and activate the digestive system. Intact whole grains that are not cracked before cooking are a source of water-soluble fiber.

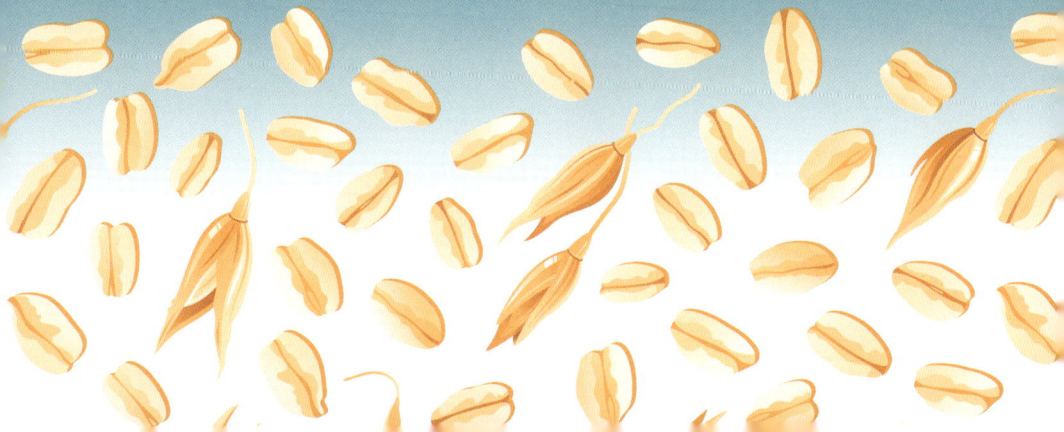

Eat Nuts and Seeds

Nuts and seeds are healthy choices for combatting fatigue and hunger.
Eating a variety of nuts and seeds in your diet provides healthy nutrients
and energy. Eating raw, unsalted versions is recommended. Try these:

◊ Almonds
◊ Brazil nuts
◊ Cashews
◊ Hazelnuts
◊ Pecans
◊ Walnuts
◊ Sunflower seeds
◊ Pumpkin seeds.

Nuts and seeds are perfect for a mid-afternoon snack, but the fat content
adds up quickly so watch how many you eat.

Think of five ways to incorporate more nuts into your daily diet, such as
adding them to yoghurt, using them as snacks, and so on.

1. _____

2. _____

3. _____

4. _____

5. _____

Nuts: The Longevity Link

Nuts are packed with heart-healthy monounsaturated and polyunsaturated fats, essential to long-term health. They help reduce LDL ("bad") cholesterol while boosting HDL ("good") cholesterol, lowering the risk of cardiovascular disease—a leading factor in healthy aging.

They're also rich in plant-based protein, fiber, and micronutrients such as magnesium, vitamin E, selenium, and folate, which support muscle maintenance, brain function, and immune resilience over time. Many nuts, such as walnuts, provide alpha-linolenic acid (ALA), a plant-based omega-3 fatty acid linked to reduced inflammation and improved cognitive health.

Research, including large cohort studies, consistently associates regular nut consumption with lower rates of chronic conditions including type 2 diabetes, certain cancers, and metabolic syndrome. Their combination of satiating fats, fiber, and protein can help maintain a healthy weight—another key factor in longevity.

The eating patterns in longevity-focused diets often feature nuts as a daily staple. Just a small handful (about 1–2 ounces) can provide lasting energy and vital nutrients, making nuts an easy, portable, and delicious habit for anyone aiming to live well—and live long.

Add Chia Seeds

Chia seeds contain the kind of carb content, healthy fats, and fiber that provide prolonged energy. Two tablespoons of chia provide about 11.9 grams of carbs and 5.05 g of omega-3s, which are also heart healthy and anti-inflammatory. In one study, athletes who consumed a sports gel with chia seeds reported an enhanced ability to take in and use oxygen during physical activity, improving their overall performance. For a boost of energy, sprinkle in a few tablespoons of chia seeds into your morning smoothie or add a scoop to your afternoon yogurt.

Eat More Lean Protein

Studies suggest that high consumption of processed red meats (such as bacon, sausages, and deli meats) is associated with an increased risk of heart disease, certain cancers, especially colorectal cancer, and type 2 diabetes. There's also evidence that it leads to chronic inflammation, oxidative stress, and the buildup of harmful compounds like advanced glycation end-products.

Compared to higher-fat cuts of meat or heavily processed proteins, lean sources—such as poultry, fish, eggs, low-fat dairy, and plant-based proteins like beans or lentils—tend to be lower in calories and saturated fat, which can reduce the risk of cardiovascular disease. A diet rich in lean protein can also help regulate blood sugar levels and support healthy weight management, lowering the likelihood of type 2 diabetes and obesity, both of which can shorten lifespan.

What lean protein sources do you currently enjoy or feel curious to try, and how could you realistically include them in your weekly meals?

If you replaced one less nutritious food each day with a lean protein option, what would you choose, and how might that change how you feel physically and mentally?

What barriers might make it hard for you to eat more lean protein, and what small, practical steps can you take to overcome them this week?

_____

_____

_____

_____

_____

Live Leaner, Live Longer

Two recent studies suggest that increasing plant protein intake in place of animal protein may lower the risk of premature death. In a study published in 2020, in The BMJ, Harvard and Tehran University researchers pooled data from 32 studies involving over 715,000 participants, with follow-ups ranging from 3.5 to 32 years. They found that replacing 3 percent of total daily calories with plant protein sources (such as beans, nuts, and whole grains) was associated with a 5 percent reduction in all-cause mortality risk.

The second study, published in 2020, in *JAMA Internal Medicine*, followed more than 416,000 adults (ages 50–71 at baseline) for 16 years. Replacing 3 percent of calories from animal protein with plant protein was linked to a 10 percent lower risk of death from any cause. Substituting plant protein for eggs and red meat showed the largest benefit—up to a 24 percent risk reduction in men and 21 percent in women, particularly among those with higher egg and red meat consumption.

Song, M., & Satija, A., et al. (2020). Plant protein intake and all cause and cause specific mortality: Prospective cohort study and meta-analysis of cohort studies. *The BMJ*, 370, m2412. https://doi.org/10.1136/bmj.m2412

Huang, J., et al. (2020). Association of animal and plant protein intake with all-cause and cause-specific mortality. *JAMA Internal Medicine*, 180(9), 1173–1184. https://doi.org/10.1001/jamainternmed.2020.2790

Stay Hydrated

Because it slows circulation and makes your heart work harder to pump oxygen to the brain and the rest of the body, dehydration can cause energy dips that leave you feeling sluggishness and unable to focus. Research has found that being as little as 2 percent dehydrated impacts attention and hand-eye coordination.

Most of us don't drink sufficient water. According to the Institute of Medicine and National Academies of Sciences:

◊ The average woman should consume approximately 11.4 cups (2.7 liters) of water (that includes in beverages and food) every day to stay hydrated.

◊ The average man should consume about 15.6 cups (3.7 liters) of water (that includes in beverages and food) every day to stay hydrated.

Try these tips to help you stay hydrated:

◊ Drink a glass of water before each meal

◊ Keep a refillable water bottle with you throughout the day

◊ Use a straw to make it easier to drink

◊ Start your day with a big glass of water

◊ Add lemon, herbs, or pieces of fruit to your water to make it flavorful

◊ Drink milk, unsweetened juice, tea, or coffee to boost water intake.

If you are dehydrated, consider adding an occasional electrolyte tab to your water. Water with electrolytes can help hydrate cells faster than plain water alone. Do not drink water or other liquids in excess, as that can cause negative health effects.

Are you currently drinking sufficient amounts of water each day? If not, list three ways you can boost your water consumption and commit to doing so.

1. _____

2. _____

3. _____

Water is Life

Adequate hydration is a cornerstone of healthy aging. Water is essential for nearly every physiological process: regulating body temperature, delivering nutrients to cells, flushing out waste, lubricating joints, and maintaining healthy skin. Chronic mild dehydration can strain the kidneys, thicken the blood, and contribute to fatigue, brain fog, and reduced physical performance—factors that, over time, can erode overall health.

Recent research from the National Institutes of Health has linked optimal hydration to healthier biomarkers and lower risk of chronic diseases, including heart disease, lung disorders, and even premature death. Proper fluid intake supports cardiovascular efficiency, helps regulate blood pressure, and aids digestion—systems that must remain robust for long-term vitality.

Staying well-hydrated may also slow aspects of biological aging. Adequate water intake helps maintain healthy sodium levels in the blood, which, when chronically elevated, are associated with increased risk of age-related conditions.

While individual needs vary, a general guide is about two to three liters daily from beverages and water-rich foods. Listening to thirst cues, monitoring urine color (pale yellow is ideal), and increasing intake during activity or heat can ensure your hydration habits are longevity-friendly.

Drink Caffeine Wisely

We all know that a boost of caffeine makes you feel more awake and alert. Many find it improves focus, but caffeine's half-life is around three to five hours, which means that half of the caffeine will be gone from your body within a few hours after you drink it. That said, caffeine's effects can last up to seven hours, so you may want to avoid it in the evening, particularly if you are having trouble sleeping.

Products that contain caffeine include:

◊ Coffee

◊ Tea

◊ Fizzy drinks

◊ Energy drinks

◊ Some painkillers and herbal remedies.

Coffee, in particular, has been shown to have many health benefits, but moderation is key.

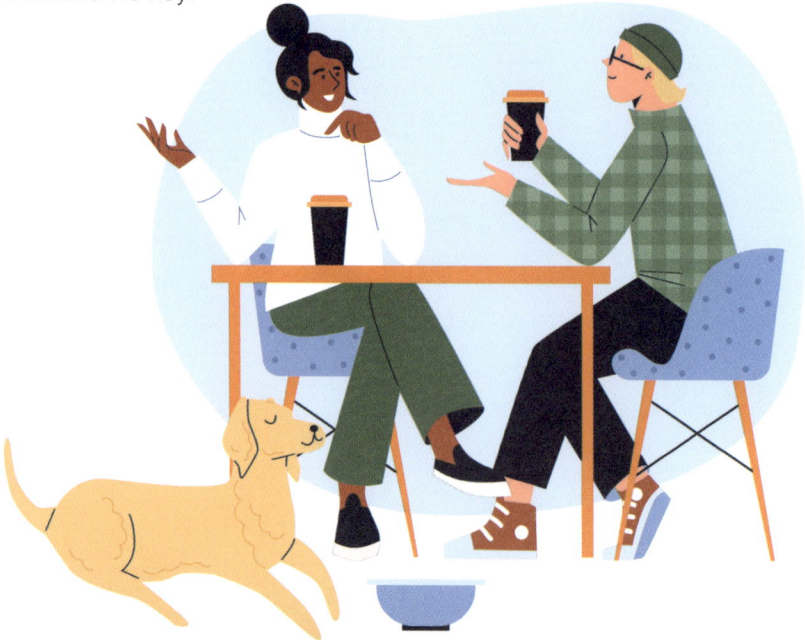

Drink Your First Coffee Around 10:30 am

Levels of the hormone cortisol (which, among other fuctions, regulates the body's energy) typically peak between 8 am and 9 am, which is why you often feel most energetic in the early morning. Research suggests that if you drink coffee during this peak hour, the caffeine's energy-boosting, mood-lifting effects won't be nearly as effective as waiting until your cortisol levels drop, which happens for most people between 9:30 am and 11:30 am. If you time your coffee break around 10:30 am, you'll maximize its energizing effect.

Try White Tea

White tea typically goes through less processing and has a delicate flavor that requires little sweetening. It also has the highest concentration of L-theanine, an amino acid that stimulates alpha brain waves to boost alertness, while also producing a calming effect. And because a cup of white tea contains less caffeine (15 milligrams) than other teas (up to 50 mg) and coffee (120 mg), it's more hydrating, which also helps boost and sustain energy.

Sip Green Tea

While it's never a good idea to drink large amounts of caffeine in the afternoon, small doses can provide just the right amount of lift that won't keep you up at night. A cup of green tea has less caffeine that coffee or black tea and contains the compound L-Theanine, which helps promote relaxation and balances out caffeine jitters.

Exercise

Exercise

Your body is more than just the vehicle for your brain. Once you start inhabiting it, paying attention to it, nurturing it, and moving it, you'll soon recognize how powerful your body can be, and how much capacity you can generate to for better brain function and to live longer and better.

Kerry J. Stewart, professor of medicine and director of clinical and research exercise physiology at Johns Hopkins University School of Medicine, trumpets the benefits of exercise in boosting both physical and mental energy. "Exercise has consistently been linked to improved vigor and overall quality of life," he reported in a 2023 WebMD article. "People who become active have a greater sense of self-confidence. But exercise also improves the working efficiency of your heart, lungs, and muscles, which is the equivalent of improving the fuel efficiency of a car. It gives you more energy for any kind of activity."

Exercise can lift both the physical and mental fatigue that many experience in a busy modern life. University of Georgia researchers found that sedentary people who complained of fatigue were able to increase their energy levels by 20 percent and decrease their fatigue by 65 percent by engaging in regular, low-intensity exercise, according to a 2008 study. Study author Patrick J. O'Connor, a professor of kinesiology at UGA, attributes the energy boost to "exercise-induced changes in activity in brain neurons and circuits that underlie feelings of energy and fatigue. It's likely that neurotransmitters like norepinephrine, dopamine and histamine are part of the process."

Exercise is a natural energy booster, because whenever you do it, oxygen-rich blood surges through your body to your heart, muscles, and brain. Even if you can spare only ten minutes, regularly squeezing a workout into your day will help keep your energy levels at their peak. Move around every chance you get, even if it's just to pace while you're on the phone. Exercise also positively impacts sleep which, in turn, boosts energy levels.

Exercise doesn't have to involve trips to the gym. It can be as simple as any of these activities:

◊ Standing or walking during work meetings

◊ Taking the stairs instead of the elevator

◊ Parking farther away and walking

◊ Scheduling 'active time'

◊ Walking during your lunch break

◊ Walking while on phone calls instead of sitting

◊ Pacing while thinking

◊ Gardening

◊ Dancing to music while doing chores

◊ Fidgeting such as tapping feet, shifting in your seat (yes, it burns calories)

◊ Biking to nearby errands instead of driving.

◊ Walking to the mailbox instead of stopping by in the car

◊ Carrying laundry up and down stairs.

◊ Stretching while watching TV

◊ Balancing on one foot while brushing teeth

◊ Taking the long way inside stores or offices.

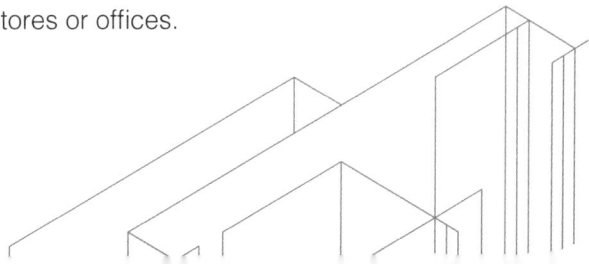

Lift weights or roll out the exercise ball. Climb a few flights of stairs at lunch and jog after dinner. To add an extra kick to your workout, breathe deeply for your first one or two minutes of cardio. Simply inhale from your belly; then breathe out slowly, imagining you're pulling your navel toward your spine.

Exercise not only boosts your energy, but it boosts your mood, too. Exercise releases endorphins that contribute to greater feelings of well-being and a 'natural high.' So, when you're feeling a little low on energy, don't skip that gym session, as you could be missing out on impressive mental and energy gains.

What are five ways you can incorporate more exercise in your daily life, starting now?

1. _____

2. _____

3. _____

4. _____

5. _____

What are some of your hang ups about exercise? What do you think are the roots of these hang ups and have you tried to overcome them?

_____

_____

What kind of exercise or movement do you enjoy? What prevents you from doing it more?

_____

_____

Get 150 Minutes at a Minimum

Getting 150 minutes of moderate physical activity each week is recommended for long-term health. These minutes can be divided throughout the week to be more manageable, but keep in mind that people who exercise regularly have fewer blood sugar spikes, which affects how energetic they feel. Moderate exercise can be anything from brisk walking to swimming, or even a game of pickleball. Cycling and resistance training also do the trick. If you've not exercised for a while, start slow and ramp up each week. For example, begin by slow walking and keep increasing your speed and distance until you're able to walk briskly for longer periods of time.

Start with a schedule that feels manageable. Over time, as your body adapts, you can increase intensity, duration, or the number of sessions. The key is consistency and gradual progression to avoid injury. Listen to your body. Rest and recovery are essential parts of any workout routine. If you feel overly fatigued or experience discomfort, don't hesitate to scale back or take an extra rest day. Life happens, and sometimes you may need to shift your workout days or duration. That's OK! The key is to stay committed to the overall routine and find ways to adapt when needed.

"If you don't make time for exercise, you'll probably have to make time for illness."

Traditional Saying

My Exercise Commitments

Create an exercise schedule (choose which day, which time of day, and what exercise you will choose) and then commit to a minimum of 150 minutes of moderate physical activity each week.

What do you think you commit to? Use this space to map out your commitment.

_____

_____

_____

_____

_____

_____

_____

_____

_____

_____

_____

_____

_____

_____

Easy Brain-Boosting Exercise Ideas

Take a Power Walk

Need a quick power surge? According to a 2012 study from Northern Kentucky University, a fifteen-minute walk can make a difference, whether you're out in nature or on a treadmill. Note, however, that if you want to rest as a means of restoring energy, they found that resting outdoors in nature is more effective than remaining indoors to rest.

Walk in Sunshine

Research suggests that just a few minutes of walking outside on a warm, clear day may enhance mood, memory, and the ability to absorb new information. Going outside can even improve your self-esteem. If you absolutely can't get out, at least open the shades and soak up some sun. Remember, if you take that walk shorty after waking up, it will boost your energy even more!

Ride a Bike

Riding a bicycle often provides a marvelous opportunity for sunlight to boost your serotonin, but whether you ride inside on a stationary bike or outside, the physicality will quicken your heartbeat and expand blood vessels to let more blood flow through your veins and thereby boost and distribute energy. Spending ten to fifteen minutes on the bike will give you the boost you need to tackle the rest of the day and help you achieve a better night's sleep. Consider using a bike to commute or run local errands.

Go for a Light Jog

You don't have to jog long distances or at a fast pace to boost your energy. Simply moving your legs will help you feel more awake, pump adrenaline throughout your body, increase your heart rate and blood circulation, and energize and prepare you for the next obstacle.

Move More, Live Longer

Recent studies of participants using fitness trackers that around 7,000–8,000 daily steps seems to hit a 'sweet spot' for lowering your odds of dying early. Even 'weekend warriors' who cram their exercise into just one or two days can still see significant health gains compared to couch-bound peers.

The longevity boost isn't just for the young. Massive global cohort studies confirm that staying active well into your seventies and eighties still pays off, with lower risks of heart disease, cancer, and premature death. Intensity matters. Workouts that raise your heart rate deliver extra cardiovascular perks. But the takeaway is refreshingly doable: small, consistent increases in movement make a big difference. Even swapping the elevator for stairs, or walking while you talk on the phone, can add up to more healthy years.

Inoue K, Tsugawa Y, Mayeda ER, Ritz B. Association of Daily Step Patterns With Mortality in US Adults. *JAMA Netw Open.* 2023;6(3):e235174. doi:10.1001/jamanetworkopen.2023.5174

Martinez-Gomez D, et al. Physical Activity and All-Cause Mortality by Age in 4 Multinational Megacohorts. *JAMA Netw Open.* 2024;7(11):e2446802. doi:10.1001/jamanetworkopen.2024.46802

"The body benefits from movement, and the mind benefits from stillness."

Sakyong Mipham

Practice Yoga

Yoga may be more than a tool for stress relief: it could also be a contributor to a longer, healthier life. Its blend of physical postures, breathing techniques, and meditation supports multiple systems that influence healthy aging.

Physically, yoga improves strength, flexibility, and balance, reducing the risk of falls and mobility loss as we age. Its gentle, low-impact nature makes it accessible across decades of life, helping preserve muscle mass and joint health without overstraining the body. Regular practice also supports cardiovascular fitness, circulation, and respiratory capacity, all vital for longevity.

On the mental and emotional front, yoga's emphasis on mindfulness helps regulate the body's stress response. Lower chronic stress translates into reduced inflammation and lower levels of cortisol, both of which are linked to decreased risk of age-related diseases such as hypertension, diabetes, and heart disease.

Studies have also shown that yoga can improve sleep quality, cognitive function, and emotional well-being, factors strongly correlated with long-term health. In many longevity-focused cultures, movement practices that integrate body and mind are central to daily life. Yoga offers a modern, adaptable version of that principle, helping practitioners move, breathe, and age with grace.

Although almost any exercise is good, yoga may be especially effective for the mind-body connection. After six weeks of once-a-week yoga classes, volunteers in a British study by the National Health Service reported improvements in clear-mindedness, energy, and confidence. It also works no matter your age. In 2006, University of Oregon researchers offered yoga instruction to 135 men and women ages 65 to 85. At the end of six months, participants reported an increased sense of well-being, a boost in overall energy, and improved mental clarity.

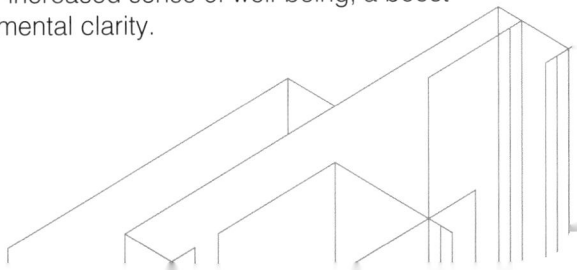

Easy Pose or Sukhasana

This simple sitting pose is designed to help you feel more grounded and less stressed out. Place a yoga mat or cushion on the floor and sit cross-legged on it. Place your hands around each knee with your palms facing upwards and each thumb and forefinger forming a circle. Straighten your spine and wiggle your bottom until your spine is perfectly aligned with your hips. As you inhale, imagine lifting your chest toward the sky, and, when you exhale, feel the release of breath grounding you through your hips. While breathing normally, hold this pose for three to five minutes. Release your legs and move to the next position.

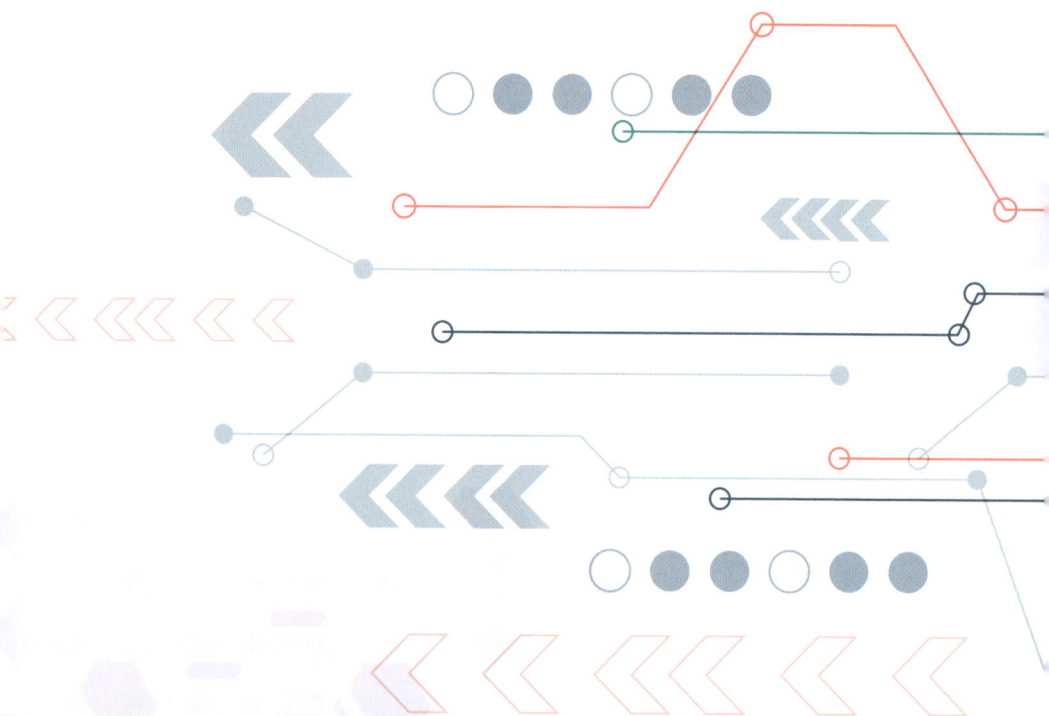

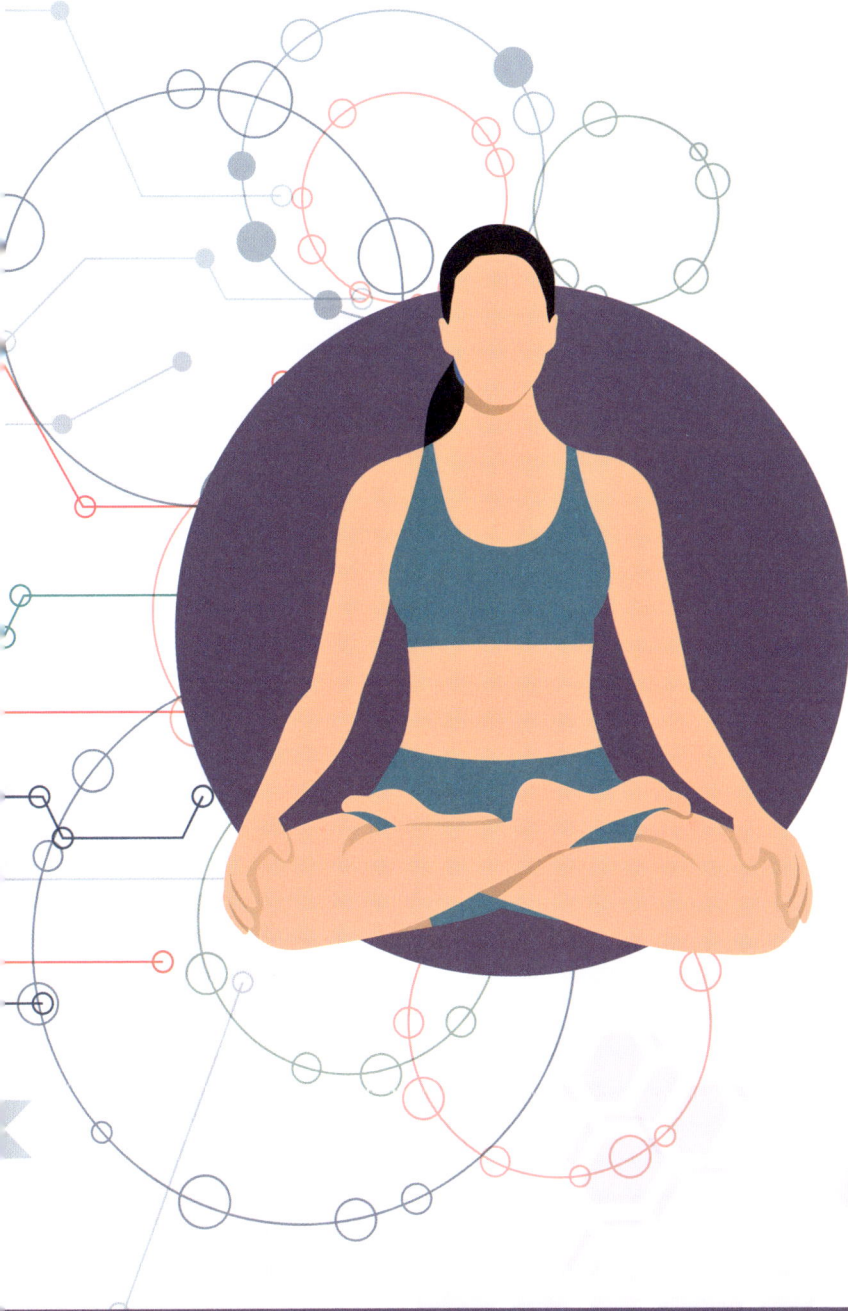

Upward-Facing Dog or Urdhva Mukha Svanasana

To stimulate your spinal cord and soothe your parasympathetic nervous system, lie face down on your yoga mat with your feet hip-width apart and the tops of your feet pressing against the mat. Place your hands beside your abdomen, palm down, with your fingers pointed toward the top of the mat. Inhale and push your upper torso up, lengthening your arms completely and pressing down through your palms. Lift your torso upward and distribute your weight so your hands and your hips hold you in balance. Puff out your chest and rotate your shoulders back. With your upper back extended breathe for thirty seconds to one minute, then slowly lower your upper torso. To release, lift until you are resting your buttocks on your feet then move to a sitting position.

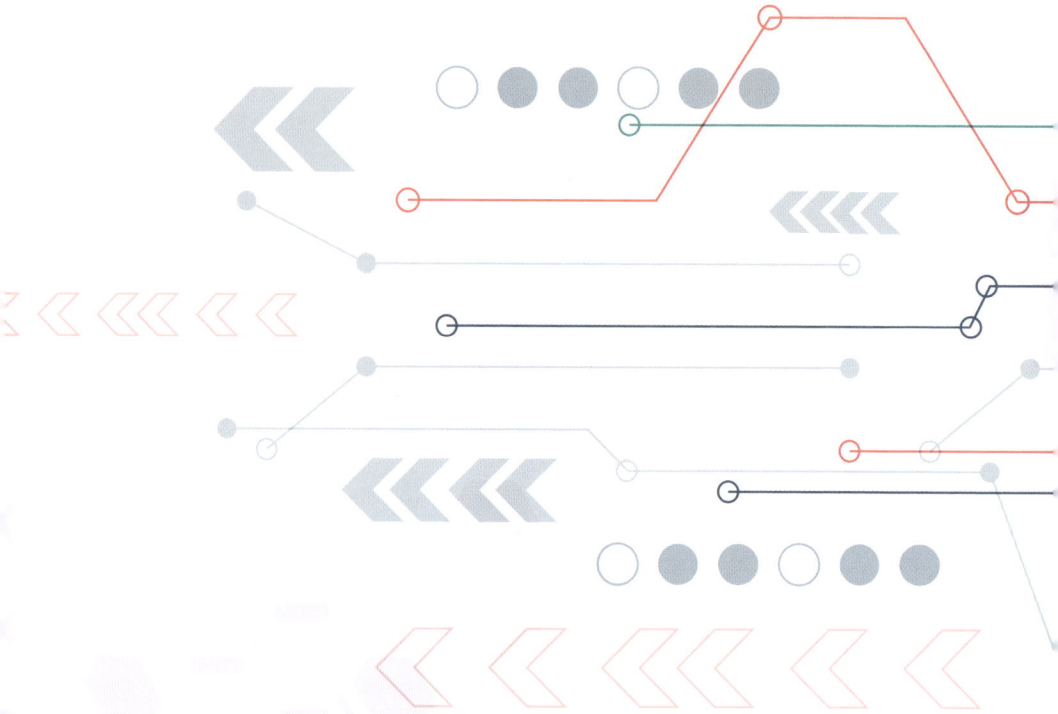

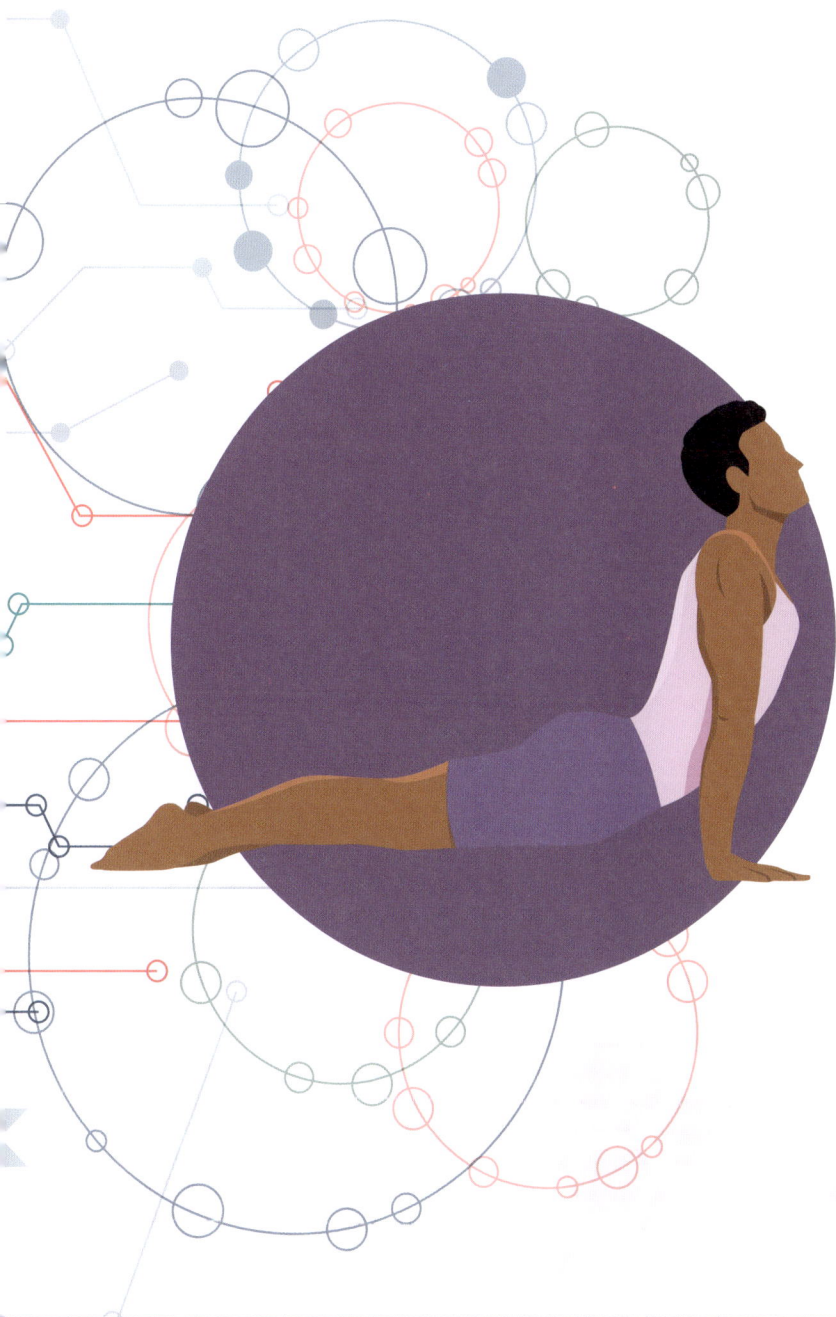

Forward Bend or Uttanasana

To further lengthen and release tension in your spine, as well as stimulate your nervous system, bring your arms down your body while bending forward, from your hips—not your waist. Bring your hands to the mat, lining up your fingertips with your toes, then press your palms flat to the mat—or use blocks to shorten the distance—while keeping your knees straight, or softly bent but not locked. While holding the pose: with each inhalation, lift and lengthen your front torso just slightly, and, with each exhalation, release a little more fully into the forward bend. Hold until you're no longer comfortable. To come up, inhale and place your hands onto your hips. Press your tailbone down and contract your abdominal muscles as you slowly rise.

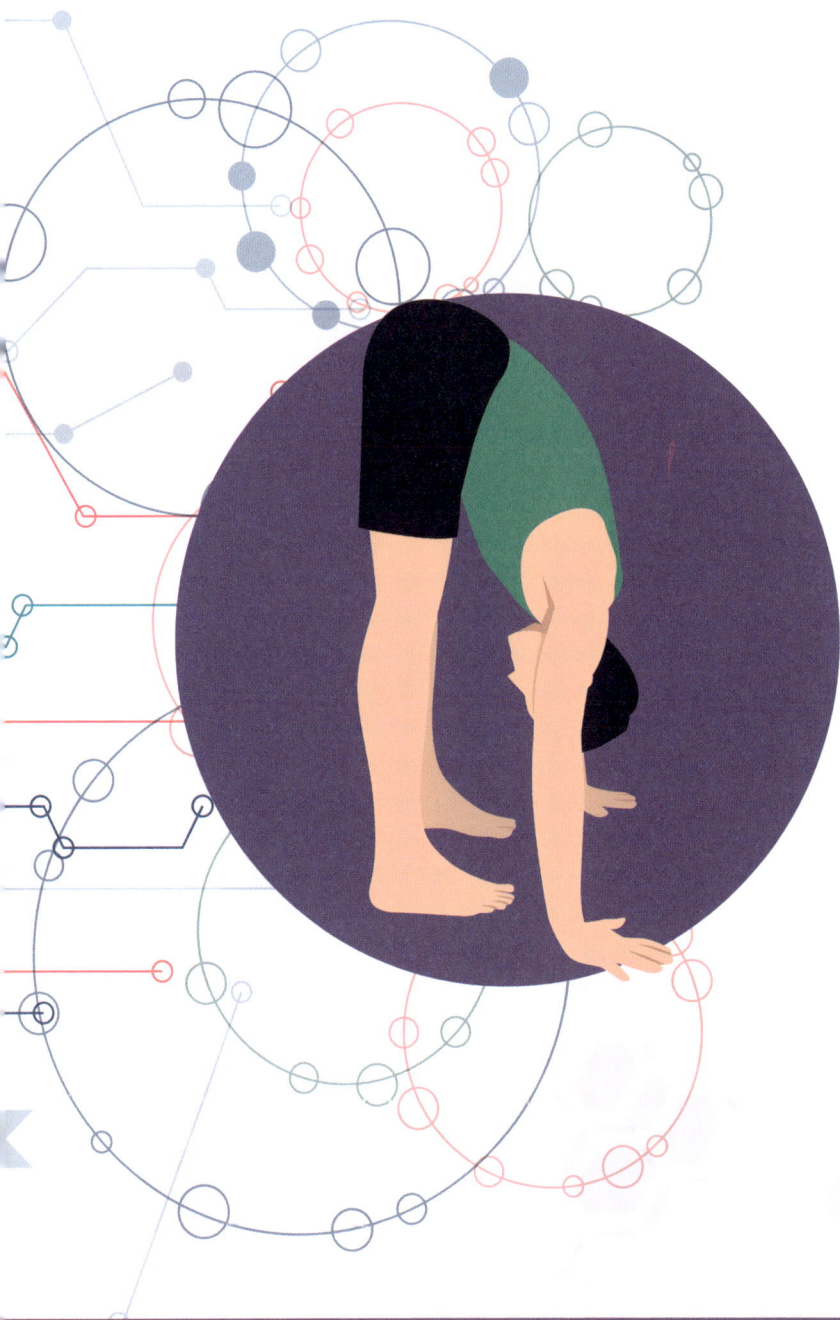

Child's Pose or Balasana

This pose simulates a mother holding her child, relaxing and breathing deeply in it provides a sense of calm, comfort, contentment, and safety. Begin by kneeling on the floor, then bring your big toes together and sit on your heels. Separate your knees to align with your hips. Exhale and lean forward from your hips, positioning your torso between your thighs. Move your hip bones outward to lengthen your tailbone and tuck your chin slightly to lift the base of your skull to stretch the back of your neck. You can either walk your hands toward the front of your mat or reach backwards toward your feet to rest your arms alongside your torso—palms up. Once in position, release your shoulders toward the floor. Since this is a resting pose, you should be comfortable holding it for five minutes or so while breathing normally. To come up: first lengthen your front torso, then, with an inhalation, lift from your tailbone as it presses down and into the pelvis.

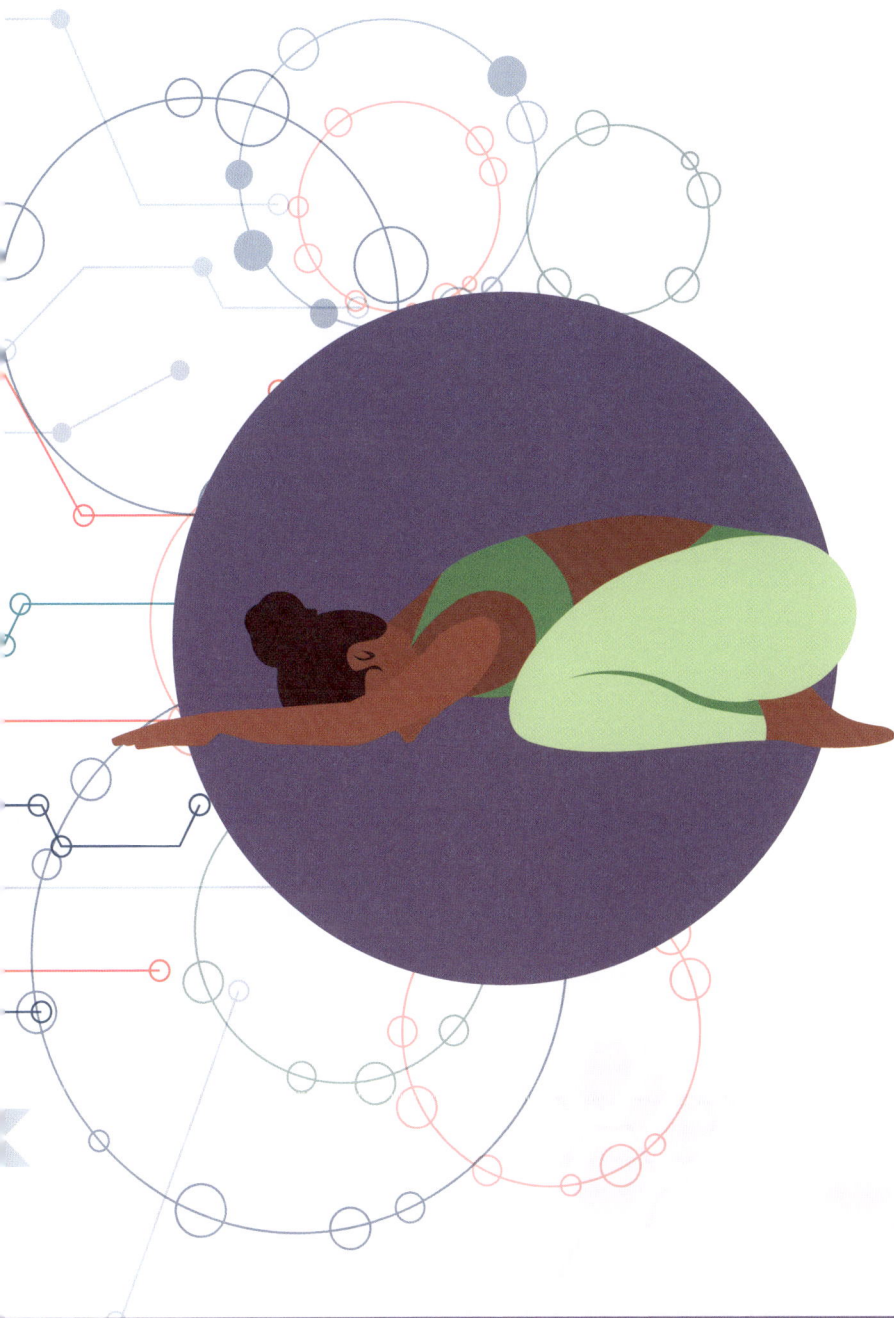

Corpse Pose or Savasana

This is the resting pose typically done at the end of a yoga session. It's designed to release all tension, clear your mind, and refresh your body. For this pose, lie down on your back then straighten and separate your legs. Place your arms alongside your body, slightly separated from your torso, with palms upwards but relaxed, allowing your fingers to curl in. Tuck your shoulder blades in for more back support. Once you're in position, relax your whole body—including your face. Lie still and breathe naturally while keeping your mind free of thoughts. Some people like listening to gentle music and setting a timer to help with focus but simply noticing your breath and the quiet is also relaxing. Work toward staying in this pose for ten minutes. To come out, while keeping your eyes closed, slowly deepen your breath, wiggle your fingers and toes, then gradually raise your arms overhead and stretch upwards from your hands and downward from your feet. Bring your knees to your chest, roll over to one side, then use your bottom arm as a pillow and pause for a moment curled into a fetal position. After a few breaths, use your hands to lift you back to a sitting position.

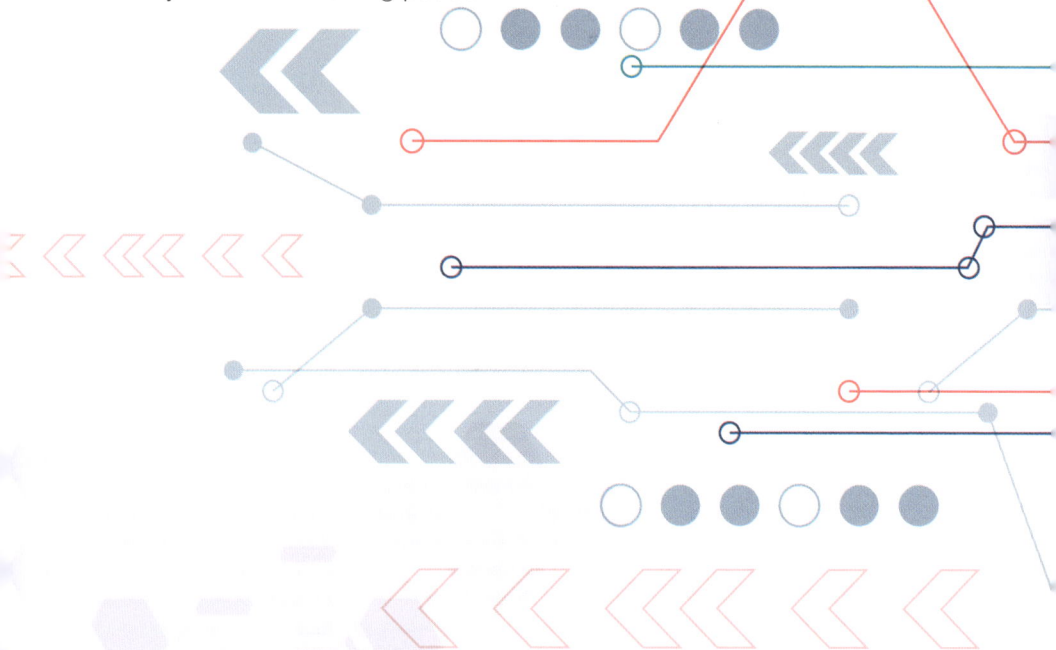

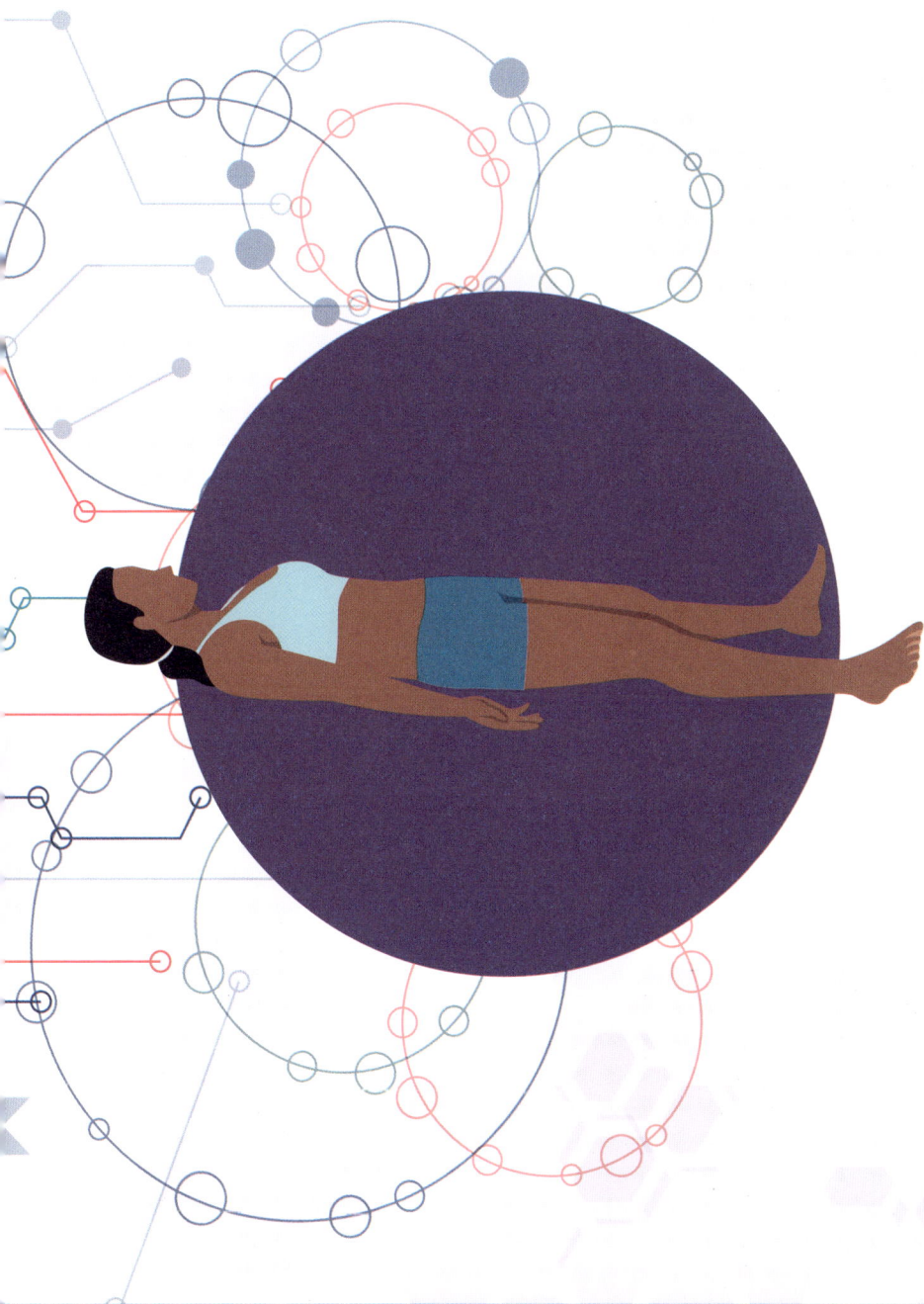

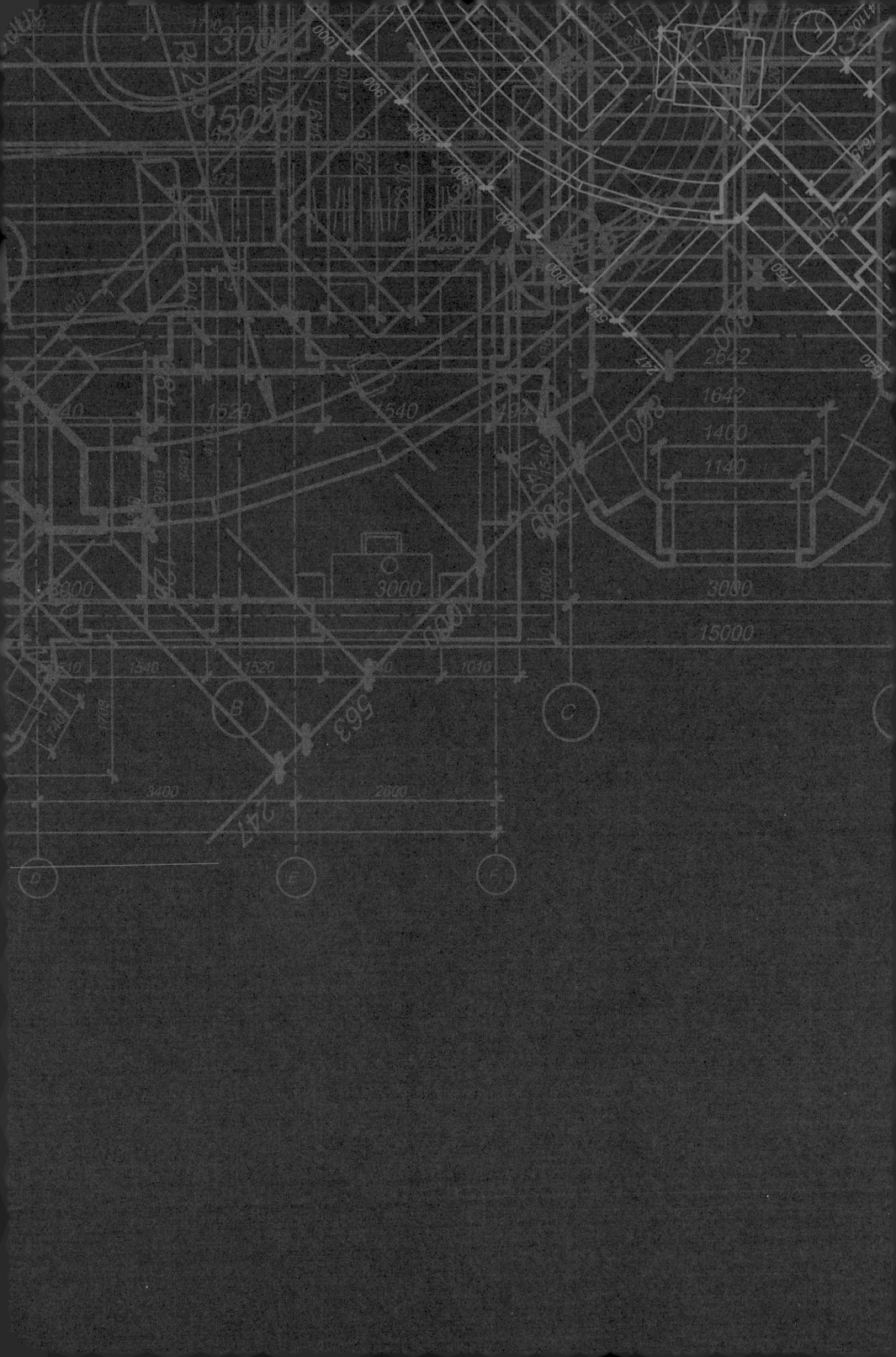

Sleep

Sleep

"The blue light that's outside in the early morning gives you a natural energy boost, no caffeine required! Blue light turns off melatonin production and turns on wakefulness."

Molly Maloof, MD

Sleep is crucial for optimal brain and physical function. It plays a central role in cognitive processes such as memory consolidation, learning, and emotional regulation. During sleep, the brain clears waste products accumulated throughout the day, including beta-amyloid, a protein linked to Alzheimer's disease. This 'cleaning' process, known as the glymphatic system, helps maintain long-term brain health.

Sleep also strengthens memories. In the stages of deep sleep (slow-wave sleep) and REM (rapid eye movement) sleep, the brain consolidates and processes information learned throughout the day, converting short-term memories into long-term storage. Without sufficient sleep, the brain's ability to retain and recall information diminishes, impairing learning and cognitive performance. Sleep has a direct impact on neuroplasticity, your brain's ability to incorporate and integrate the input it receives. When you sleep well, it is easier for you to learn and to remember. A poor night of sleep can negatively impact your ability to retain information. For your brain to problem-solve, make decisions, and even to access its source of creativity, you need quality sleep.

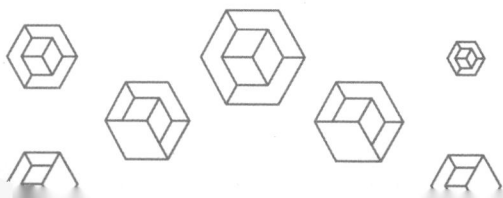

Quality sleep is a vital, and often overlooked, ingredient for a long, healthy life. During deep and REM stages, the body repairs tissues, consolidates memories, and regulates hormones that control appetite, stress, and immune function. Chronic sleep deprivation disrupts these processes, increasing the risk of heart disease, diabetes, obesity, depression, and cognitive decline—all of which can shorten lifespan.

Research suggests that consistently getting seven to nine hours of restorative sleep is associated with lower mortality risk and better overall health. Poor sleep, on the other hand, elevates inflammation and blood pressure, accelerates cellular aging, and impairs the brain's ability to clear toxins.

Sleep quality matters as much as duration: a dark, cool, quiet environment, a regular bedtime, and limited caffeine or screen time before bed all support better rest. Simply put, making sleep a priority is one of the most powerful, natural longevity tools we have.

Sleep also supports emotional stability by regulating hormones such as cortisol and serotonin. Lack of sleep can lead to increased stress, irritability, and mood swings, while adequate rest promotes emotional resilience. In short, sleep is not a passive state but an active process vital for mental clarity, memory, emotional balance, and overall brain health. Given all this, it's easy to see why sleep is essential to cognitive health. To understand how you can improve your sleep for better cognition, it's important to understand the sleep cycle.

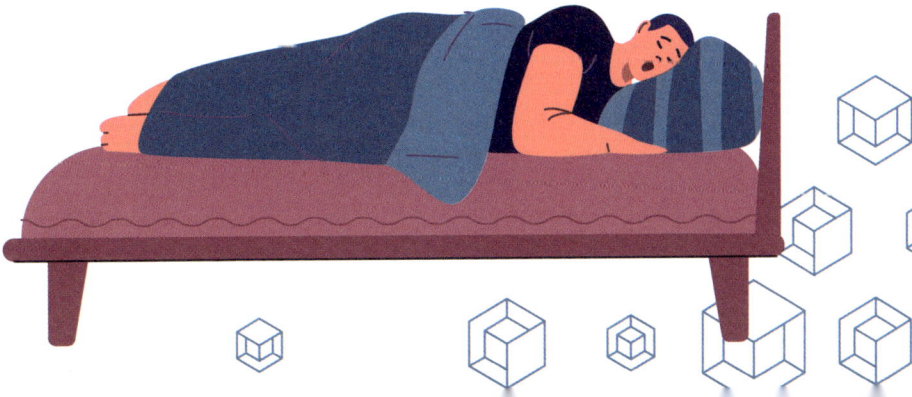

The Sleep Cycle

A typical sleep cycle consists of four stages. During an average night of sleep, you continue to go through this cycle as many as four or five times. As the cycle continues to repeat itself, you spend more time in the fourth stage—REM Sleep—and less time in the third stage—Non-REM Deep Sleep. If you are sleeping well throughout the night, you will not experience the first stage of the sleep cycle again after the first full cycle has been completed.

It is important to note that the sleep cycle does not always occur sequentially. Typically, you will cycle through the first three stages, then back to the second, and then you'll jump to the fourth. As the cycles go on, you may occasionally skip the third or fourth stage in a given cycle.

Stage One: Falling Asleep

This Non-REM stage of the sleep cycle is when you transition from wakefulness to sleep. The duration of this stage is usually less than ten minutes. During this time, your heartbeat, breathing, eye movements, and brain waves begin to slow down. Your muscles will start to relax and you may feel your muscles twitch.

Stage Two: Light Sleep

This is another Non-REM stage of sleep. This light sleep stage lasts around twenty minutes and will repeat throughout the evening as you continue to go through the sleep cycle. About 50 percent of your total time sleeping each night occurs in this stage. Your heartbeat and breathing slow down further. Your muscles continue to relax more deeply, your body temperature drops, and your eye movements stop. Your brain waves also continue to slow down, but they may be interrupted by short bursts of electrical activity known as sleep spindles. These sleep spindles are thought to assist with the sorting and processing of memories. Scientists believe this is the role of a sleep spindle because an increase in sleep spindle activity occurs the night after someone has learned a lot of new information.

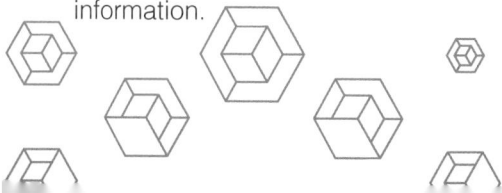

Stage Three: Deep Sleep

The final Non-REM stage of sleep consists of the deep sleep you need to feel fully rested. During this sleep stage, your muscles are fully relaxed and your heartbeat and breath reach their lowest levels. Your brain waves slow down and your brain consolidates things you learned that day. During deep sleep, your body physically repairs itself, releases hormones for bone and muscle health and growth, and strengthens your immunity.

Stage Four: Dream Sleep

During this stage of REM sleep, your eyes move from side to side while your eyes are closed. This cycle occurs about 90 minutes after falling asleep and continues to repeat throughout the night. Your heart, blood pressure, breathing, and brain waves come close to matching their waking levels. Your arm and leg muscles are paralyzed to keep you safe while you dream. Though dreaming can occur in other stages of sleep, most dreams occur during the REM stage. As you age, your REM cycles become shorter.

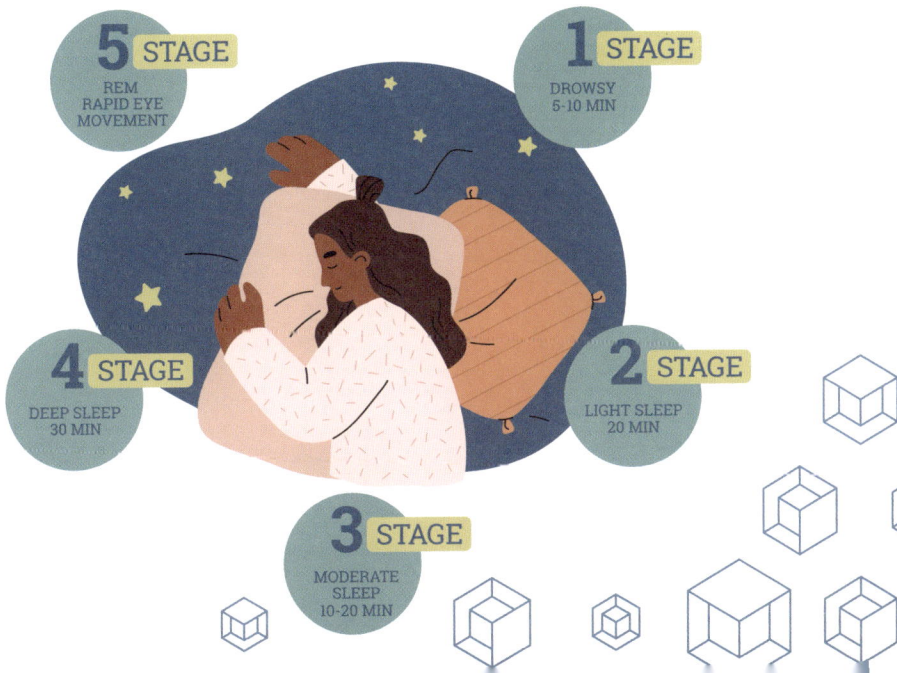

How Much Sleep Do You Need?

According to Orfeu Buxton, an associate professor of biobehavioral health at Pennsylvania State University, a panel of over a dozen sleep experts reviewed previous sleep studies and "agreed that an adult needs a minimum of seven hours of sleep to achieve optimal cognitive, emotional, and physical health."

If you're sleeping less than seven hours at night, Buxton recommends moving up your bedtime by ten-minute increments each night until you hit the seven-hour mark.

Studies also show that starting your day at the same time each day, helps regulate your circadian rhythm (see page 61-63), otherwise known as your body's clock. Establishing a routine of waking up and going to bed around the same time daily—and adhering to it, even on weekends and vacations—will improve your sleep.

How many hours are you currently sleeping at night?

_____

_____

_____

_____

Do you feel refreshed upon awakening?

_____

_____

_____

_____

Circadian Rhythm

Your circadian rhythm is a 24-hour cycle connected to your internal clock, regulating important processes for your body, such as appetite, hormones, and sleep. You can think of your circadian rhythm as a piece of your internal programming connected to a teeny-tiny clock inside of your brain that, when calibrated correctly, keeps all the systems in your body running at the appropriate time. This teeny-tiny clock is located in the *suprachiasmatic nucleus*, or SCN, which is found in the hypothalamus in your brain. This internal clock is calibrated using a variety of factors, but the most influential is light. Your body's internal clock sets itself by recognizing the difference between light and darkness from signals sent to your brain by your eyes.

When your circadian rhythm is synced correctly, lightness—or daylight— causes your body to enter an energetic state by releasing a hormone known as cortisol. On the flip side, darkness—or nighttime— causes your body to release melatonin, a hormone that aids in sleep. When your circadian rhythm is off, you may not be able to fall asleep or stay asleep, and you may feel disoriented or sluggish during the day.

"Sleep is not an optional lifestyle luxury. Sleep is a non-negotiable biological necessity."

Matthew Walker

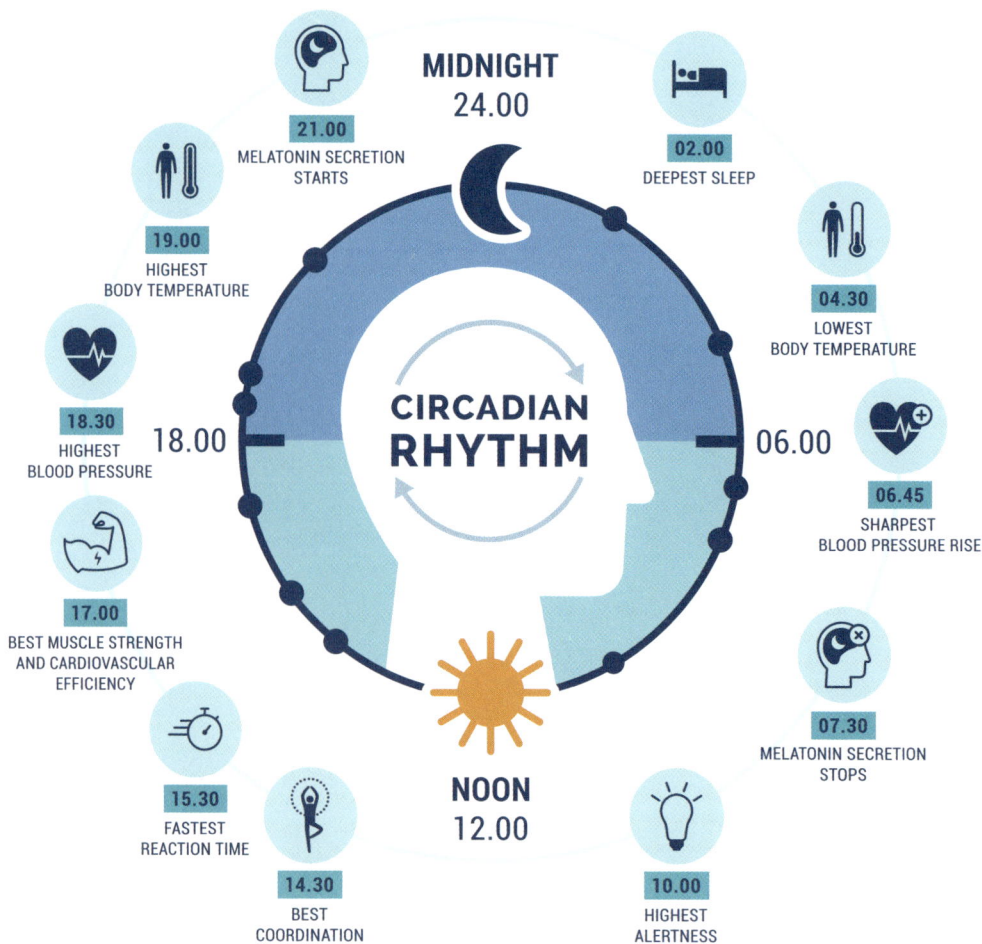

MIDNIGHT
24.00

21.00
MELATONIN SECRETION
STARTS

02.00
DEEPEST SLEEP

19.00
HIGHEST
BODY TEMPERATURE

04.30
LOWEST
BODY TEMPERATURE

18.30
HIGHEST
BLOOD PRESSURE

18.00

CIRCADIAN
RHYTHM

06.00

06.45
SHARPEST
BLOOD PRESSURE RISE

17.00
BEST MUSCLE STRENGTH
AND CARDIOVASCULAR
EFFICIENCY

07.30
MELATONIN SECRETION
STOPS

15.30
FASTEST
REACTION TIME

14.30
BEST
COORDINATION

NOON
12.00

10.00
HIGHEST
ALERTNESS

Circadian Rhythm Balancing Exercise

If your circadian rhythm is out of calibration, you can experience drowsiness and fatigue during the day and an inability to fall asleep and stay asleep at night. You can reset your circadian rhythm by completing the following exercise. You may find this exercise is balancing for you because it creates a routine that gets you outside to breathe in fresh air and connect with nature. If you enjoy it, you can turn this exercise into a part of your daily life.

◊   Commit to a period of time between three and 14 consecutive days. The longer you incorporate this practice, the more consistent and predictable your circadian rhythm will become.

◊   Look up the timing for sunrise and sunset. Set your schedule. For each day of the exercise, set an alarm or a reminder on your phone (you can use your phone's calendar app to do this), for 10 minutes before sunrise and sunset.

◊   Rise with the sun. When your morning alarm goes off, get up and go outside. Find a comfortable position, sitting or standing, and watch the sunrise. Turn your face towards the sun. Sit outside for ten minutes after the sun has risen.

◊   Screens disappear when the sun sets. When your evening alarm goes off, turn off all screens in your home. Turn off televisions, computers, phone, or any screen that emits light. For greater impact, you can also dim or minimize the other sources of artificial light in your home. Go outside, turn your face towards the sun, and watch the sunset. Sit outside for 10 minutes after the sun has set.

◊   Repeat. Do this each day for the time period you identified in step one.

Bonus Points

If you want to make this exercise even more effective, do not take a nap while you are resetting your internal clock. Also, aim to go to bed around the same time each night to deeply calibrate your body.

Practice Good Sleep Hygiene

According to sleep scientists, creating and fostering a certain atmosphere for sleeping can play a significant role in how well you sleep well and whether you wake feeling energized. Although this has nothing whatsoever to do with your bed linens or cleanliness, it's called sleep hygiene. Sleep hygiene describes the quality of your sleep environment. To improve your sleep hygiene, consider the following.

Sleep in a fully dark bedroom. Absolute darkness helps you fall asleep and stay asleep. It bolsters your body's circadian rhythm and prevents any signs of light from telling your body it's time to wake up. Use block-out curtains and even banish nightlights or, if the display light gives off too much light, turn your alarm clock away from you.

Keep the room cool. A comfortable temperature helps your body transition into a restful state and tend to what it needs to do while sleeping, such as restoring your brain. Also, if you get either hot or cold during the night, it tends to disturb your sleep. Sleep experts have determined that a temperature around 65°F (18.3°C) is ideal for optimal sleep.

Use white noise (a fan or quiet music) to fall asleep and stay asleep. Low-volume background noise can help induce sleepiness. It can also tamp down any outside noise and even quiet any ringing in your ears. Try sounds that feel soothing, such as ocean waves.

Avoid artificial light before bedtime. Light from cell phones, computers, televisions, and other electronics may impair your circadian rhythm. Put them down at least one hour before bedtime. Get in the habit of not using them in your bedroom at night.

Some scientists recommend that you only use your bedroom for sleeping and dressing. Reading in bed may feel pleasurable, but they recommend that you read in another room and only slide into bed when you're ready to sleep. Over time, this alerts your body that you are readying yourself for sleep, which will help it transition from wakefulness to sleep.

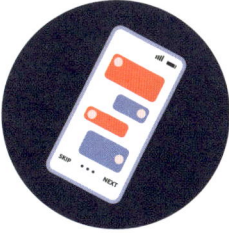

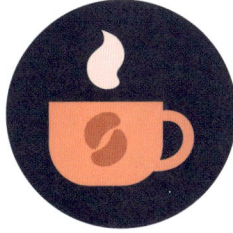

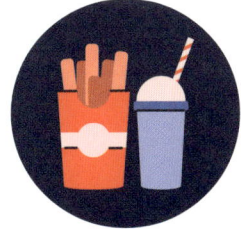

Sleep Hygiene Checklist

◊ Avoid screens (phone, tablet, TV) at least 1 hour before bedtime .

◊ Avoid caffeine or stimulants after mid-afternoon

◊ Engage in relaxing pre-sleep activities (reading, meditation, gentle stretches)

◊ Go to bed and woke up at consistent times, even on weekends

◊ Kept the bedroom cool, dark, and quiet

◊ Avoid heavy meals or alcohol within 2–3 hours of bedtime

◊ Limited naps during the day, especially late afternoon or evening

◊ Use the bed only for sleep and intimacy (no work or screen time)

◊ Practice deep breathing or mindfulness exercises before sleeping

◊ Reduce noise with earplugs or white noise if necessary

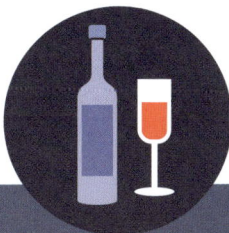

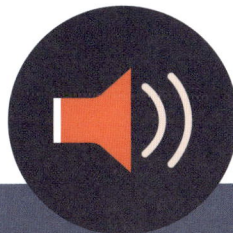

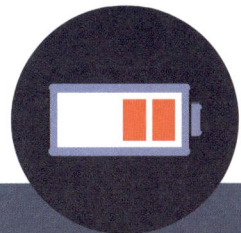

Establishing a Bedtime Routine

A bedtime routine or ritual can go a long way toward improving your sleep hygiene. As you are looking to set up a routine, or ritual, incorporate elements that are soothing, relaxing, calming, and signal a feeling of peace and safety so that you can gently drift off to sleep. Think about the things you already do each night before bed. Consider ways you can improve upon those things and identify practices you would like to add to your ritual.

For example, if you currently brush your teeth each night and take off your makeup using a makeup wipe before bed, assess this. When you brush your teeth, could you improve the process by investing in a better toothbrush? Could you swap out your evening toothpaste for something more calming like an herbal toothpaste with chamomile? Instead of using a makeup wipe could you spend an extra minute or two taking off your makeup a different way that is better for your skin and more calming? Those are the kind of questions you will want to ask yourself to ensure that you have created the very best wind-down ritual or bedtime routine possible. Following are different suggestions to include in your bedtime ritual.

> "Eat healthily, sleep well, breathe deeply, move harmoniously."
>
> Jean-Pierre Barral

A Relaxing Bathing Ritual

Though a hot shower feels great, it can also be too stimulating before bed. Choose a temperature that Goldilocks would approve of: not too hot and not too cold. It should feel slightly warmer than the temperature of your skin. You can light a candle or play calming music. Use soothing products with aromatherapy benefits. A tingly citrus body wash or scalp invigorating shampoo is great during the day, but these stimulating products negatively impact your ability to relax.

Instead, think about owning a set of daytime and nighttime products with varying scents. Nighttime products can include soothing, earthy, calming, and relaxing scents.

A shower is a time for you to clean your body and mind. As you wash away the physical debris of the day, visualize the mental debris of the day—stress, anxiety, negative emotions, or overwhelm —rinsing away with it. Take deep cleansing breaths while you do this. Tell yourself that anything negative that you experienced that day has been washed down the drain. You can even say it aloud at the end of your shower: "I am clean and clear both in body and mind. I am ready to rest and restore." Invest in a soft robe and slippers to put on the moment you have finished drying off.

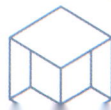

Your Morning Routine

Water is a wonderful element to incorporate into your morning ritual to signal to your body that it's time to engage with the day. If you are not someone who likes to shower first thing in the morning, you can still use water in your routine. Go to your sink and run some cold water. Splash it on your face a few times. Gently pat your face dry.

If you are someone who enjoys a morning shower to start the day, there are two types of showers you can try: cold and invigorating. These two types of showers can also be combined.

If you are new to cold showers, give yourself time to acclimate to the idea. You can take a normal shower and finish off with a short burst of cold water as you are getting started. Work up to thirty seconds. Then work up to a minute. Eventually, get yourself to the point where you can endure—and even enjoy! —a 2 to 3-minute cold shower.

Once you are at the point where you are ready to start your day with a cold shower—and no warm water to ease into it—you can let your body adjust by first running your hands and feet under the water and then taking a few deep breaths before stepping in. Do not hold your breath during the shower. Instead, breathe deeply, allowing the oxygen in your lungs and the cool water on your skin to energize you.

Cold showers have many health benefits. Starting your day with a cold shower makes you alert and helps you feel fresh and awake. It also boosts your immune system, decreases stress, and aids in weight loss. There are added beauty benefits to cold showers—they are less drying than hot showers, so your hair and skin will appear healthier and more hydrated. Additionally, cold showers have been shown to reduce the symptoms of depression.

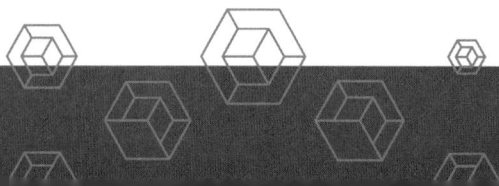

If you create a routine, or ritual, for your morning, you can stretch your sleep benefits even further. A routine is, by definition, something predictable. This predictability allows your brain to relax, as it does not need to engage in any critical thinking. The presence of a morning routine allows your brain to wake slowly and naturally.

If a cold shower isn't for you, or if you choose to start with a warm shower and then finish with a cold shower, then you will enjoy an invigorating shower specifically designed for the morning hours. Use invigorating products with aromatherapy benefits. If you are using products such as body wash, shaving cream, shampoo, and conditioner, consider purchasing some products that are specific to your morning routine. Think of scents that you find invigorating and fresh: citrus, mint, and bright florals all work. If you would like to make your own scent, you can purchase unscented products and give them a boost with some of your favorite brightly scented essential oils. You can also soak a sponge in eucalyptus or lemon oil and place it in your shower for added aromatherapy benefits.

Using Visualization to Fall Asleep Faster

Visualization is an especially powerful practice when you are seeking sleep. The process of focusing on something lovely engages your brain, while simultaneously relaxing it. This allows your mind to stop engaging with the stressors of the day, to focus on something beautiful, and to soothe itself to sleep.

Visualizations should be done after you are ready for bed, are comfortably tucked in, and have your eyes closed.

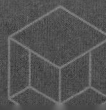

Empty Room Visualization

Visualize yourself in an empty room. This room has nothing on the walls and no furniture in it. Even though the room is bare, you feel overwhelmingly safe and calm in the space. Nothing can hurt you. Nothing can interfere. This is your special space.

Imagine a large cozy chair appearing in the room. Visualize yourself sitting in this chair. You feel how comfortable it is against your body. You feel completely supported. Spend some time relaxing in this chair and breathing deeply.

Now imagine a big window appearing on one of the walls that your chair is facing. It fills almost the entire wall. You can sit in your comfortable chair feeling safe in your special space, but you can now look outside. The vista that you are looking at is the most beautiful you have ever seen. There are fields of flowers swaying softly in the breeze as far as the eye can see. Pink and purple clouds move slowly across the sky. The sun's rays are gently shining as it begins to set.

Sit and observe this landscape from the comfort of your chair. Feel free to change the landscape at any time. This is your visualization. You can visualize a tropical beach or snowy mountain peaks or a peaceful lake. All you have to do is visualize something that you find beautiful and imagine it in as much detail as possible. Do this for as long as you need to prepare yourself for sleep or until you fall asleep.

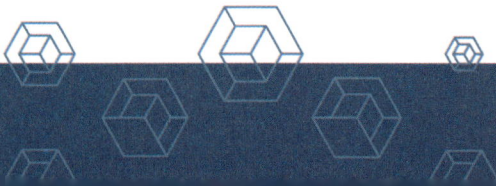

Starry Night Visualization

Visualize yourself lying on your back in a large, beautiful field at night while looking up at the stars. Imagine a warm night- time breeze comfortably grazing your skin.

Now focus on that sky full of stars. Visualize more stars than you have ever seen. The stars are bright, clear, white pinpricks of light scattered across the inky sky. Some dots of light are brighter and bigger than the others. These stars are closer to you. Other stars are small and harder to see. These stars must be very far away.

Visualize a meteor shower beginning. Shooting stars begin to appear, one at a time. Slowly at first and then with increasing frequency. Notice each shooting star. Notice the bright white trail of shimmer that it briefly leaves behind before it seems to be absorbed into the dark of night. Allow yourself to observe the incredible beauty of this.

Wish on the shooting stars. As you continue to watch the shooting stars, you remember that some people believe you should "wish upon a shooting star." Begin to wish, earnestly and from your heart, for all the things you desire on each star you see. Know in your heart of hearts that all these wishes will come true. After all, who has ever been blessed with such a meteor shower before? Do this for as long as you need to prepare yourself for sleep or until you fall asleep.

Lazy River

Visualize yourself sitting in an inner tube in a very peaceful lazy river. The water is comfortable on your skin.

Allow yourself to float gently down the river. As you begin to float, slowly and safely down the river, it occurs to you that you have nothing more to do than enjoy the feeling of the water on your skin and the beauty of the nature around you.

Imagine looking around and noticing the clear water and the lush banks. You notice deer approaching the river with you in it with no fear and drinking from the pure water. You see trees and flowers, birds and bunnies, soft rays of sunshine and blue sky. You take your time to feel grateful for each of these things.

As you continue to float, a white butterfly joins you. This butterfly continues with you down the river. The butterfly is not afraid of you and wants to experience the path of your floating journey by flying around you. You watch the butterfly leave your side, only occasionally, to perch on one of the countless colorful flowers on the river's edge and then to join you again as you float down the river. Do this for as long as you need to prepare yourself for sleep or until you fall asleep.

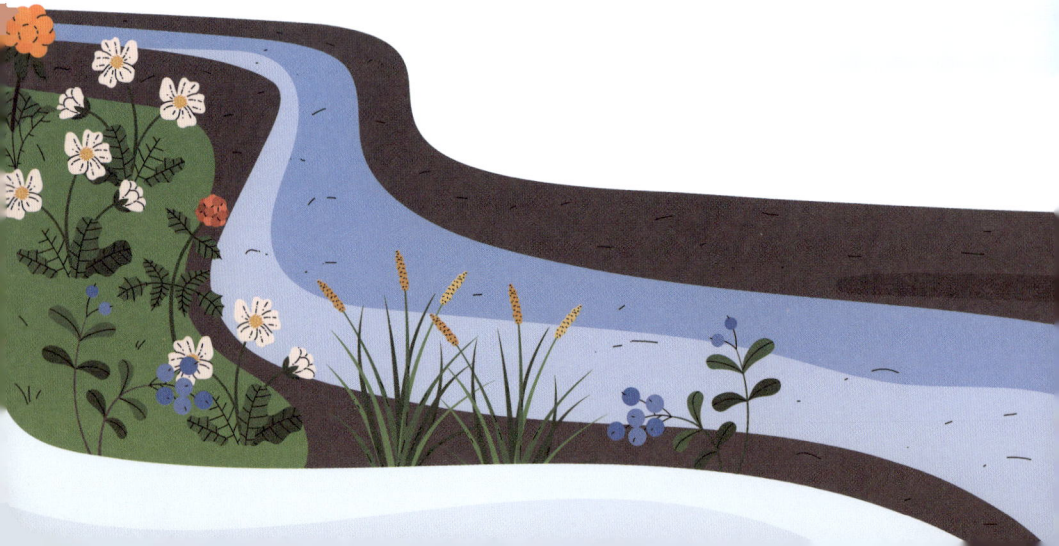

Floating on a Cloud

Once you are comfortable in bed, close your eyes, and take deep breaths that start from your belly and up through your nose. Hold for each for moment, then exhale slowly through your mouth. With each breath, allow your body to relax more deeply.

Now, picture yourself lying on a gentle cloud, supporting you perfectly. Your body feels weightless until it feels like you are actually floating above it. You begin to float.

As you float, you're surrounded by the most peaceful sense of freedom. The air around you is the perfect temperature. You glance beneath you and see the earth in perfect harmony. You are not afraid. You are part of it. You're filled with an inner sense of calm.

The cloud sways slightly in rhythm with your breathing. As you continue to float, your tension melts away. Your body is completely relaxed, your mind calm and clear. Allow yourself to drift into a peaceful state. You don't have a care in the world.

The sun sets gently and you are surrounded by the stars, one with them, free of any earthly burdens.

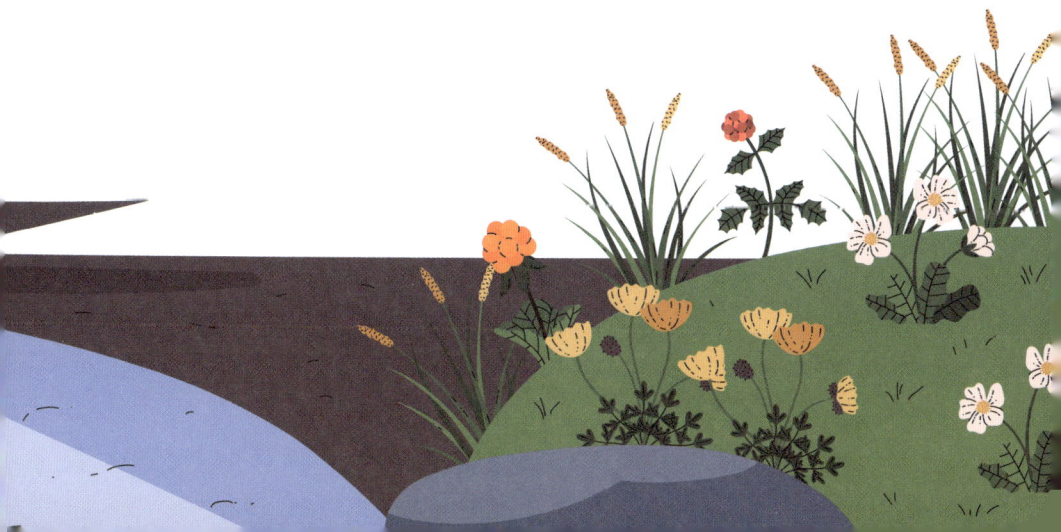

Waking Up and Starting Your Day

You've probably heard that how you start your morning can determine your success for the day. So, what are the best ways to get your day going? Here are a few methods to consider.

The Natural Method

The natural method of waking involves relying on your body's circadian rhythm (see pages 61-63). If you are going to sleep and waking at relatively the same time each day and you are controlling your exposure to unnecessary light in the evening, this method might be the one you prefer.

This method involves going to sleep at your designated bedtime and trusting that your body will wake at the appropriate time after receiving an adequate amount of sleep. This might sound impossible, but you've likely experienced it before. Have you ever woken up a few minutes before the alarm you set is supposed to go off? Or have you ever accidentally forgotten to set your alarm and woken up at the correct time anyway? These things happen because your body's circadian rhythm instinctively knows when to wake.

The Light Method

The light method takes the natural method and gives it some circadian rhythm signaling assistance. Light is one of the key factors that influences your circadian rhythm's sleeping and waking functions. Using light strategically can signal to your brain that it is time to wake up. It is also a smooth transition from sleeping to waking because the gradual increase in light will also allow a gradual transition to waking.

You can influence your circadian rhythm by exposing yourself to light in the morning in a variety of ways.

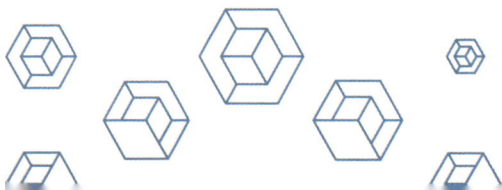

Leave the Blinds Up

You can leave your blinds up if you live in an area that isn't influenced by artificial external light. For example, if you live in the country, this method might be great for you. However, if you live in the city, your circadian rhythm will be disrupted by the artificial city lights. If you live in an area where you can do this, leave the blinds open so that the sunrise in the morning wakes you up. Note: this can be difficult for some people when the moon is bright, as this keeps some people up. Pay attention to your individual sensitivities.

Timer-Controlled Blinds

For those willing to invest in their sleep habits, this option is a great one. There are blinds available that can be controlled by your smartphone and smart home devices. You can assign different times for closing and opening or lowering and raising the blinds. For blinds to be synced with your circadian rhythm, close the blinds completely after sunset. Many of these are also blackout blinds, so you will not have light interrupting your period of sleep. Time the blinds to open about 10 minutes before sunrise. This way, the natural increase in light that occurs during sunrise will assist you in waking.

Light-Waking Device

For less money than automated blinds, you can purchase a bedside device that uses light to wake you. You set your desired waking time and the device will begin to emit light, first very dim light that gets increasingly brighter light the sunrise, to wake you naturally by your desired time. For those who feel nervous trusting their waking times to light and light alone, this is a good option because most of these devices have a backup alarm that sounds if the light does not wake you.

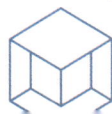

The Alarm Method

If you are one of countless people who choose to wake using an alarm, let's look at ways that you can optimize your waking method. Think about the style of alarm you are using. If you are using an old-fashioned alarm that uses a beeping sound or radio music to wake you, throw it out. There is nothing natural, gentle, or soothing about a loud robotic beeping noise or the static of a radio station.

Your cell phone might not be serving you. Keeping your cell phone in your bedroom exposes you to blue light, it emits harmful radiation that is typically near your head as you sleep, and many of the sounds included on the phone as alarm choices are not pleasant noises in the morning, or ever. If you must keep your cell phone in the bedroom and use it as an alarm, place it on the other side of the room. This way, you are not as close to the harmful radiation or blue light and you will have to walk across the room to wake up. Also, upgrade your alarm sound. Download an app with alarm sounds that are pleasing, like ambient music or nature sounds. If you would like to use an alarm to wake, try investing in a bedside alarm clock made specifically for gentle waking. There are many alarm clocks on the market with a large library of waking sounds and even clocks that consider different kinds of waking. For example, you might be someone who likes to wake up and still lie in bed for a few minutes. You might want an alarm clock that allows you to set two separate alarms, the first with a very gentle sound and the second with a slightly more impactful sound to get you out of bed. Some of these alarm clocks even have sleep sounds and guided meditations and breathwork practices on them for an added nighttime benefit. Additionally, many of today's alarm clocks have a blackout mode that allows you to stop all light emitting from the device while you sleep.

If you feel nervous that you're going to not wake up on time or that you're going to miss something important, set a backup alarm. Once you have established a regular sleeping pattern with predictable sleeping and waking times, your body will begin to know what to do, but the backup alarm can gently assist. Your backup alarm should be set for thirty minutes after your goal waking time. If your body does not alert you to wake, your alarm will. While you are training your body to wake naturally, add a 30-minute buffer to your morning just in case you have to rely on that backup alarm.

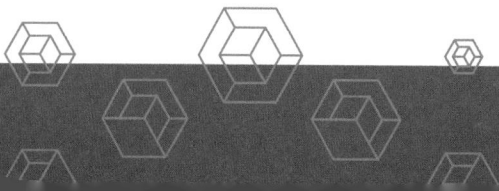

The Power of the Slow Start

Once you're awake, don't feel the need to jump out of bed. Allow the sleep you just experienced to really sink in. Feel free to stretch and move a bit before you get out of bed.

Once you are ready to leave your bed, you can continue to enjoy the last remnants of your sleep by extending the cozy feeling. You can designate a zone near your bed to store some comfortable items that you can put on first thing. Invest in some comfortable slippers and a robe for yourself. Your robe can be flannel for extra warmth, cotton for ease and breathability, or something like silk or satin for a luxurious start to your day. Keeping yourself cozy allows you to continue to wake up gradually as your circadian rhythm begins to release cortisol to assist you with waking fully. Once you have covered your feet in your slippers and wrapped your body in your robe, you can begin your morning routine.

Take a Power Nap

If you're sleeping well at night, a brief midday snooze can be an excellent pick-me-up. For most people, keeping your nap short (around 30 minutes) is ideal. Longer naps lead into REM sleep, which can leave you feeling drained rather than restored. The exception would be for people who work extremely long hours, who could nap for 90 minutes, when needed. The National Institute of Mental Health found that short afternoon naps improved cognitive function, especially alertness.

Here are some tips for power napping:

◊　Don't nap too late in the day; aim for mid-afternoon, around 3 pm
◊　Set a soft alarm for 30 minutes
◊　Use an eye mask or ear plugs to block out distractions.

Sleep Tracking

Tracking your sleep can provide valuable insights into your overall health and cognitive functioning, enabling you to optimize your rest and improve daily performance. Here are some key reasons why you should track your sleep.

1. Identify Sleep Patterns

Tracking sleep helps you recognize patterns, such as the time it takes to fall asleep, how often you wake up during the night, and the duration of deep sleep versus light sleep. These patterns can reveal whether you're getting restorative rest or if your sleep quality needs improvement.

2. Improve Sleep Quality

Many people focus on sleep duration without considering quality. Tracking allows you to monitor how much deep (slow-wave) and REM sleep you get, which are crucial for memory consolidation, emotional regulation, and cognitive performance. Identifying disruptions or irregularities in these stages can guide you to make lifestyle or environmental changes to enhance sleep quality.

3. Optimize Health and Well-Being

Poor sleep is linked to a range of health issues, from impaired cognitive function and memory to increased risk of chronic conditions like heart disease and diabetes. By tracking your sleep, you can spot trends and make changes to improve your overall health, such as adjusting your bedtime routine, reducing caffeine intake, or managing stress.

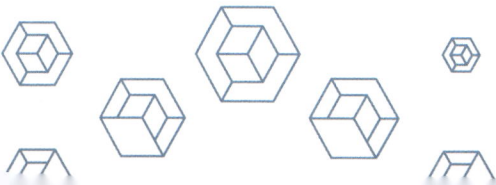

4. Boost Cognitive Function

Tracking sleep helps you assess whether you're getting enough restful sleep to improve focus, memory, and mental clarity. By understanding your sleep patterns, you can adjust your habits to maximize cognitive performance during the day.

5. Identify Sleep Disorders

If you notice consistent disruptions, such as waking up frequently or feeling unrested despite adequate hours of sleep, sleep tracking can help identify potential sleep disorders like sleep apnea, insomnia, or restless leg syndrome. Early detection allows you to seek medical advice and receive appropriate treatment.

6. Motivation and Accountability

A sleep tracker provides tangible data that can motivate you to improve your habits. Whether through tracking the time spent in bed or monitoring the effectiveness of new sleep strategies, it creates accountability and encourages you to prioritize rest as part of a healthy lifestyle.

Use the trackers on the following pages to keep track of your sleep progress to make connections between sleep improvement and your cognitive functioning.

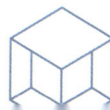

Sleep Tracker

DATE

WHAT I DID BEFORE I FELL ASLEEP

TIME I WENT TO BED: **TIME I FELL ASLEEP:**

WHAT WOKE ME UP DURING THE NIGHT

TIME I WOKE UP: **TOTAL HOURS OF SLEEP:**

HOW HAVE I SLEPT?

NOTES

Sleep Tracker

DATE

WHAT I DID BEFORE I FELL ASLEEP

TIME I WENT TO BED: **TIME I FELL ASLEEP:**

WHAT WOKE ME UP DURING THE NIGHT

TIME I WOKE UP: **TOTAL HOURS OF SLEEP:**

HOW HAVE I SLEPT?

NOTES

Sleep Tracker

DATE

WHAT I DID BEFORE I FELL ASLEEP

TIME I WENT TO BED: **TIME I FELL ASLEEP:**

WHAT WOKE ME UP DURING THE NIGHT

TIME I WOKE UP: **TOTAL HOURS OF SLEEP:**

HOW HAVE I SLEPT?

NOTES

Sleep Tracker

DATE

WHAT I DID BEFORE I FELL ASLEEP

TIME I WENT TO BED: **TIME I FELL ASLEEP:**

WHAT WOKE ME UP DURING THE NIGHT

TIME I WOKE UP: **TOTAL HOURS OF SLEEP:**

HOW HAVE I SLEPT?

NOTES

Sleep Tracker

DATE	

WHAT I DID BEFORE I FELL ASLEEP

TIME I WENT TO BED: TIME I FELL ASLEEP:

WHAT WOKE ME UP DURING THE NIGHT

TIME I WOKE UP: TOTAL HOURS OF SLEEP:

HOW HAVE I SLEPT?

NOTES

Sleep Tracker

DATE

WHAT I DID BEFORE I FELL ASLEEP

TIME I WENT TO BED: **TIME I FELL ASLEEP:**

WHAT WOKE ME UP DURING THE NIGHT

TIME I WOKE UP: **TOTAL HOURS OF SLEEP:**

HOW HAVE I SLEPT?

NOTES

Sleep Tracker

DATE

WHAT I DID BEFORE I FELL ASLEEP

TIME I WENT TO BED: **TIME I FELL ASLEEP:**

WHAT WOKE ME UP DURING THE NIGHT

TIME I WOKE UP: **TOTAL HOURS OF SLEEP:**

HOW HAVE I SLEPT?

NOTES

Sleep Tracker

DATE

WHAT I DID BEFORE I FELL ASLEEP

TIME I WENT TO BED: **TIME I FELL ASLEEP:**

WHAT WOKE ME UP DURING THE NIGHT

TIME I WOKE UP: **TOTAL HOURS OF SLEEP:**

HOW HAVE I SLEPT?

NOTES

Sleep Tracker

DATE

WHAT I DID BEFORE I FELL ASLEEP

TIME I WENT TO BED: **TIME I FELL ASLEEP:**

WHAT WOKE ME UP DURING THE NIGHT

TIME I WOKE UP: **TOTAL HOURS OF SLEEP:**

HOW HAVE I SLEPT?

NOTES

Sleep Tracker

DATE

WHAT I DID BEFORE I FELL ASLEEP

TIME I WENT TO BED: **TIME I FELL ASLEEP:**

WHAT WOKE ME UP DURING THE NIGHT

TIME I WOKE UP: **TOTAL HOURS OF SLEEP:**

HOW HAVE I SLEPT?

NOTES

Sleep Tracker

DATE

WHAT I DID BEFORE I FELL ASLEEP

TIME I WENT TO BED: **TIME I FELL ASLEEP:**

WHAT WOKE ME UP DURING THE NIGHT

TIME I WOKE UP: **TOTAL HOURS OF SLEEP:**

HOW HAVE I SLEPT?

NOTES

Sleep Tracker

DATE

WHAT I DID BEFORE I FELL ASLEEP

TIME I WENT TO BED: **TIME I FELL ASLEEP:**

WHAT WOKE ME UP DURING THE NIGHT

TIME I WOKE UP: **TOTAL HOURS OF SLEEP:**

HOW HAVE I SLEPT?

NOTES

Sleep Tracker

DATE

WHAT I DID BEFORE I FELL ASLEEP

TIME I WENT TO BED: **TIME I FELL ASLEEP:**

WHAT WOKE ME UP DURING THE NIGHT

TIME I WOKE UP: **TOTAL HOURS OF SLEEP:**

HOW HAVE I SLEPT?

NOTES

Sleep Tracker

DATE

WHAT I DID BEFORE I FELL ASLEEP

TIME I WENT TO BED: **TIME I FELL ASLEEP:**

WHAT WOKE ME UP DURING THE NIGHT

TIME I WOKE UP: **TOTAL HOURS OF SLEEP:**

HOW HAVE I SLEPT?

NOTES

Mental Stimulation

Mental Stimulation

Mental energy is the ability of your mind to effectively perform cognitive tasks, such as thinking, concentrating, problem-solving, decision-making, and learning. When your mental energy runs high you experience enhanced cognitive function, improved memory, and creativity. When energy reserves run low, you may experience brain fog, reduced concentration, and impaired cognitive performance.

Mental fatigue occurs when prolonged cognitive activity has depleted your brain's energy reserves. Essentially, your brain runs out of juice and starts to lag. Unlike physical tiredness, which affects your body, mental fatigue affects your cognitive functions—making it difficult to focus, make decisions, or even manage your emotions. While you can usually relieve physical fatigue by a good night's sleep or incorporating more restful moments in your schedule, mental fatigue builds over time and can become chronic. Let's discuss the emotional and physical symptoms of mental fatigue:

Emotional Symptoms of Mental Fatigue

◊ **Anxiety:** You're caught in a constant state of worry and stress

◊ **Lack of motivation:** Tasks that you used to enjoy now feel like a chore. Tasks you have to do get put off, creating more stress

◊ **Difficulty concentrating:** Your mind is so preoccupied, focusing on a single task feels out of reach

◊ **Forgetfulness:** Your brain feels like it's overloaded all the time, making it hard to eliminate or monitor distractions. This overload often leads to forgetfulness

◊ **Easily angry or irritated:** You are so tense that even small disturbances can make you lose your cool

Physical Symptoms of Mental Fatigue

◊ **Sleep issues:** It's hard to fall asleep, get the REM sleep you need, stay asleep, or wake up feeling refreshed

◊ **Physical aches:** Tension is getting stored in your muscles, leading to aches and pains, and sometimes headaches

◊ **Coping poorly:** You're using food to self-medicate by either overeating, or not eating enough to refuel

◊ **Poor food choices:** Instead of choosing food that could boost brainpower, you're indulging in sugar or fatty foods that drain brainpower

Are you experiencing any of the symptoms just described? Which ones are most concerning? Can you identify what's causing the symptoms?

_____

_____

_____

_____

_____

_____

_____

_____

_____

_____

_____

Overcoming Mental Fatigue and Stimulating Your Brain

Keeping your mind fresh and operating at optimum performance requires conscious effort. In addition to sleep, exercise, and proper nutrition, and mindfulness and meditation (see pages 130 to 173), there are several methods for overcoming fatigue and stimulating your brain.

Take Breaks and Go on Tech Fasts

Mental fatigue often results from extended periods of intense focus or concentration. To prevent this, it's important to take regular breaks. The Pomodoro Technique is a popular method where you work for 25-30 minutes, followed by a 5-minute break. After completing four cycles, take a longer break (15-30 minutes). This helps refresh your mind, maintain focus, and prevent burnout.

Constant streams of notifications and information can overwhelm our brains, making it harder to focus, process new information, or relax. Taking regular tech breaks or fasts reduces mental fatigue, stress, and information overload.

A tech fast allows the brain to rest and reset, reducing cognitive load and preventing burnout. Studies show that time away from screens helps improve attention span, creativity, and even sleep quality. For instance, the blue light emitted by devices can interfere with melatonin production, disrupting sleep patterns. By stepping away from screens, you give your body the chance to recover and reset its natural rhythms.

Tech fasts can help you to increase real-world connections, which lead to many benefits. Focusing on face-to-face interactions, engaging in physical activities, or simply spend quiet time in nature is essential to brain health.

When was the last time you took a tech break? How did you feel afterward? Use the space below to work out when and how you will incorporate this important respite into your life.

_____

_____

_____

_____

_____

_____

_____

_____

_____

_____

_____

_____

_____

_____

_____

_____

_____

_____

_____

Learn Something New

Learning something new is one of the most effective ways to stimulate your brain and promote cognitive growth. When we engage in a new activity, it kick-starts our brains' neuroplasticity. This constant reshaping of the brain enhances its ability to adapt, learn, and retain information, keeping it agile and resilient.

New experiences challenge the brain to process unfamiliar information, which activates different areas of the brain. For example, learning a new language involves memory, problem-solving, and the auditory and visual processing areas of the brain. Similarly, acquiring a new skill such as playing an instrument or learning a language stimulates multiple brain regions, including those related to fine motor control, coordination, and abstract thinking.

As we practice and repeat the new activity, the brain's neural pathways become more efficient. This repetition strengthens the connections between neurons, which leads to improved cognitive function. Essentially, the more you practice something, the more automatic and efficient the process becomes, much like building a road that is easier to travel on over time.

Furthermore, learning new things can increase the size of certain brain regions. Studies show that learning complex skills, such as juggling or making something with your hands, can lead to increased gray matter in areas associated with motor control and coordination. This growth is an indication that the brain is adapting and expanding its capabilities.

Learning something new also releases dopamine, a neurotransmitter linked to motivation and reward. This makes the process of learning enjoyable and reinforces the behavior, encouraging continued growth and engagement.

Use the space below to commit to new things you'd like to learn. Prioritize which ones are most important and consider a realistic timeline for starting and improving.

NEW SKILL	TIMELINE

Engage in Creative Activities

Creativity is a great way to recharge your brain while providing stimulation. Engaging in creative activities such as painting, writing, playing music, or even cooking can challenge the brain in new and enjoyable ways. These activities activate various cognitive functions, such as problem-solving, decision-making, and memory. Creative exercises enhance divergent thinking (thinking outside the box) and stimulate different neural networks in the brain. This can increase cognitive flexibility and help you think more clearly.

What are some creative pursuits you've long considered trying, but have been putting off? Use the space below to commit to a plan for engaging in or learning a new creative pastime.

_____

_____

_____

_____

_____

_____

_____

_____

_____

_____

Creative Pursuits That Promote Longevity

Learn a Musical Instrument - Playing instruments like the piano or guitar can improve memory and coordination.

Practice Painting or Drawing - Artistic expression stimulates brain areas related to creativity and emotion.

Engage in Pottery or Sculpture - Hands-on crafts enhance motor skills and spatial reasoning.

Write Poetry or Short Stories - Creative writing fosters imagination and cognitive flexibility.

Practice Origami - Folding paper enhances concentration and fine motor skills.

Learn Photography - Photography encourages mindfulness and creative expression.

Collage Making - Combining various materials like magazines, fabric, and photographs to create collages stimulates creativity and fine motor skills.

Calligraphy - Practicing beautiful handwriting enhances concentration and can be a meditative process, fostering mindfulness.

Digital Art Creation - Using digital tools to create art allows for experimentation with colors and designs, enhancing cognitive flexibility.

Scrapbooking - Assembling scrapbooks with personal photos and memorabilia promotes storytelling and preserves memories.

Knitting or Crocheting - These activities improve fine motor skills and can be a relaxing, repetitive process that reduces stress.

Woodworking or Model Building - Engaging in these hands-on projects enhances spatial reasoning and problem-solving abilities.

Up Your Reading Game

Reading a variety of materials is an excellent way to optimize brain function. When you read diverse types of content—fiction, non-fiction, news articles, academic papers, or even poetry—you challenge your brain in unique ways, keeping it flexible and adaptable. Reading stimulates cognitive flexibility—the ability to shift between different concepts and ideas. Fiction, for example, helps improve empathy and creativity by forcing you to understand different characters' perspectives, while non-fiction sharpens critical thinking and analytical skills. By exposing yourself to different writing styles and topics, you enhance your ability to think critically, reason, and solve problems.

Reading regularly boosts vocabulary and language skills, enhancing your communication abilities. This not only aids in understanding complex ideas but also strengthens memory and recall. The more varied your reading material, the more words, concepts, and knowledge you absorb, fostering intellectual growth.

Reading also encourages deep focus and mental discipline. In an age of constant digital distractions, sitting down to read requires sustained attention, which exercises your brain's ability to concentrate. This reinforces neural connections that support better overall brain health, memory retention, and cognitive function. All this means reading is a simple yet powerful way to keep your brain engaged and optimized.

> "Reading is to the mind what exercise is to the body."
>
> Joseph Addison

Use the space below to create a reading list you can commit to, along with a timeline for finishing it. Include books from a variety of genres.

_____

_____

_____

_____

_____

_____

_____

_____

_____

_____

_____

_____

_____

_____

_____

_____

_____

_____

_____

_____

_____

Pursue Social Relationships

Maintaining social relationships can help our brains stay engaged and enhance cognitive performance. Humans are social creatures, and our brains are wired to interact with others. Through socializing with friends, family, and colleagues, our cognitive processes are engaged, helping to maintain mental sharpness. Numerous studies have shown that social connections are linked to better cognitive function, memory retention, and overall mental health.

Meaningful conversations, problem-solving with others, and social engagement all require mental effort. When conversing, we must recall relevant information, formulate coherent thoughts, and actively listen. This kind of mental exercise helps strengthen neural pathways, improving our memory, attention, and processing speed. Regularly engaging in social interactions keeps the brain active, similar to how physical exercise keeps muscles in shape. The more we use our brains in complex, socially-driven tasks, the sharper and more flexible they become.

Social relationships also help regulate emotions, which directly affects cognitive performance. Strong relationships provide emotional support and a sense of belonging, which can reduce stress and anxiety—two factors that often impair cognitive function. Chronic stress, for example, can shrink brain structures such as the hippocampus, which is crucial for memory and learning. Positive social interactions release neurochemicals such as oxytocin, serotonin, and dopamine, which improve mood, reduce stress, and promote cognitive flexibility. In this way, having a supportive social network can mitigate the harmful effects of stress on the brain, allowing for better cognitive performance.

Social interactions often present challenges and opportunities to learn new information or develop new perspectives. Engaging in stimulating discussions, learning about others' experiences, or participating in group activities all require the brain to adapt and integrate new information. This constant learning process strengthens brain networks, particularly in areas associated with memory, problem-solving, and decision-making.

As we age, cognitive decline can become a concern. But research shows that seniors who maintain active social lives tend to experience slower rates of cognitive decline compared to those who are more socially isolated. The engagement with others helps preserve cognitive function by encouraging mental challenges and providing emotional support. Studies have also demonstrated that older adults with strong social networks perform better on cognitive tests and exhibit higher levels of brain activity, particularly in areas related to memory and executive function.

The link between socializing and brain health also extends to reducing the risk of cognitive disorders, such as dementia. A study by the University of Michigan found that individuals with strong social ties are less likely to develop Alzheimer's disease. This may be because social interaction stimulates the brain and reduces the effects of loneliness, which is considered a risk factor for cognitive decline. Loneliness can lead to depression and a lack of mental engagement, both of which are associated with a higher risk of cognitive impairment.

Use the space below to commit to five ways that you will work on improving social relationships in your life, whether it's reconnecting with people from your past, developing new relationships, or maintaining current relationships.

What are some of the barriers you encounter in maintaining social relationships? What are some of the ways you think you might be able to overcome them? Use the space below to problem solve.

_____

_____

_____

_____

_____

_____

_____

_____

List the people you interact with regularly. How do these relationships contribute to your well-being? Are there any you'd like to strengthen or expand?

_____

_____

_____

_____

_____

_____

_____

_____

_____

Think about activities or groups you'd like to join. What interests or hobbies could help you meet new people and form connections?

_____

_____

_____

_____

_____

_____

_____

_____

_____

Consider activities or groups you've always been interested in but haven't yet explored. What are some potential opportunities in your community that align with your interests?

_____

_____

_____

_____

_____

_____

_____

_____

_____

Vary Your Routine

When you introduce variety into your daily life, your brain has to adapt to changes. This adaptation requires mental effort, which strengthens cognitive functions like problem-solving, memory, and attention. A different approach to a familiar task activates regions of the brain that are involved in learning and creativity, boosting mental sharpness. Varying your routine helps combat mental fatigue and boost your energy, too. Repeating the same tasks day in and day out can lead to a decrease in motivation and focus. By adding variety, you create a sense of excitement and curiosity, which can lead to a renewed sense of purpose and energy.

Changing up your routine also promotes flexibility and the ability to deal with uncertainty—traits that are highly beneficial for mental health and cognitive resilience. The more adaptable your brain becomes, the better it can handle stress, solve complex problems, and stay engaged in daily tasks.

Shaking up your daily schedule might seem counterintuitive, but introducing variety can significantly enhance cognitive function. Engaging in new experiences stimulates neuroplasticity. Incorporating small changes, such as taking a different route to work, trying a new hobby, or altering your meal times, can activate different brain regions and improve mental flexibility. Varying daily activities is associated with better cognitive and executive functioning, as well as improved short-term memory.

> "To improve is to change; to be perfect is to change often."
>
> Winston Churchill

What is one simple action, such as taking a different route to work, trying a new hobby, or initiating a conversation, that you can take to disrupt your current pattern and bring a sense of novelty?

_____

_____

_____

_____

Visualize an ideal day that excites you. What activities would you include? How would you structure your time?

_____

_____

_____

_____

Fear often keeps us stuck in familiar but unfulfilling patterns. What's one fear (such as fear of failure, rejection, or the unknown) that has prevented you from making changes. How do you think you could confront and overcome it?

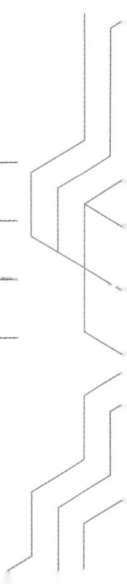

_____

_____

_____

_____

Learn and Recall One New Thing

'Novel learning,' that is learning something new, and 'retrieving' or recalling it is a technique you can easily incorporate into your day-to-day routine with a time commitment of only 10 minutes. When you retrieve information, multiple areas of your brain are engaged, including attention, language, memory. Over time, you can build up a 'cognitive reserve,' that is an ability to resist the effects of aging on your brain. Activities that involve learning new things and retrieving them later are linked to better cognitive outcomes and are more beneficial than repeating the exact same easy task every day. The combination of new learning, active recall, and use (speaking/writing) gives a stronger mental workout than passive reading. Give it a try!

Daily Novel Learning

Pick something small and novel: a new word, a fun fact, a short poem line, a recipe step, or a simple piece of trivia.
Spend 3–4 minutes learning it: read it aloud, look up a picture, or watch a 60–90s clip about it.
Close your eyes and try to recall it from memory (30-60 seconds).
Use it: write one sentence using the word/fact or tell someone about it (2–3 minutes).
At the end of the day, test yourself again (30-60 seconds). Repeat the next day with something new — but occasionally try to recall items from previous days.

Variations

Make it social: tell a friend or family member what you learned — social interaction adds extra cognitive and emotional benefits.
Pair with light activity: a short walk while practicing recall combines physical and mental stimulation (good for brain health).
Alternate words, pictures, short math tricks, mini-recipes, or a 1-minute melody. Variety helps more areas of the brain.

Seven-Day Daily Brain Booster Plan

DAY	ACTIVITY
1	Morning puzzle (crossword, jigsaw, Sudoku) for 10 minutes
2	Learn a new word or fun fact, recall it later and tell someone.
3	10-15 min of meditation or deep breathing
4	Play a game: card game, memory matching, or strategy such as chess.
5	Creative expression: paint, craft, or sketch for pleasure.
6	Listen to or sing along with music from earlier decades; optionally play a simple instrument.
7	Learn something new: a phrase in another language or another skill.

Try Brain Games and Puzzles

Mental puzzles, such as Sudoku, crossword puzzles, logic games, and memory exercises are proven to be beneficial for cognitive health because they actively challenge the brain and help you stay sharp.

One of the main benefits of solving mental puzzles is their ability to enhance problem-solving skills. Puzzles involve identifying patterns, thinking critically, and applying reason and logic. It may seem as though you're just playing a game, but these skills can transfer to real-life situations, making it easier to resolve complex problems in real time. By tackling puzzles that require varied strategies, you can train your brains to approach challenges with creativity and flexibility.

Puzzles improve memory and recall. Many mental exercises—especially memory-based games or activities that require recall of sequences or details—help strengthen both short-term and long-term memory. This can be particularly beneficial as people age, as it helps delay the onset of cognitive decline associated with conditions such as dementia or Alzheimer's disease. Crossword puzzles, for instance, challenge an individual to recall words and meanings, enhancing vocabulary retention and mental agility.

Puzzles and mental games enhance concentration and focus. You need sustained attention and the ability to block out distractions to follow through. This improved focus can lead to better attention spans in daily tasks. The brain, like any muscle, strengthens through regular exercise, and activities that require deep concentration improve the brain's ability to focus on and process complex information.

Mental puzzles can boost your processing speed. As you practice solving puzzles, you become more efficient at processing information and making decisions quickly. This can help improve reaction times and the ability to quickly assess and address situations, both in work environments and everyday life.

Finally, solving puzzles can promote neuroplasticity. With just a few minutes a day devoted to mental challenges, you can incrementally improve your brain function, and that's what bio-hacking your brain is all about!

Use this space to make a list of mentally challenging games and puzzles that you enjoy. Try the games starting on page 176 if you're looking for a place to start.

Executive Function

Mental games and puzzles can improve your executive function; that is, the cognitive processes that allow you to plan, organize, make decisions, solve problems, and regulate your behavior to achieve goals.

The core components of executive function include:

Working memory
This involves the ability to hold and manipulate information in the mind over short periods. For example, remembering a phone number long enough to dial it or keeping track of multiple instructions while completing a task.

Inhibition
This is the capacity to control impulses, resist distractions, and refrain from actions that might not be productive or appropriate. It involves delaying gratification, such as resisting the urge to check social media while working on a project.

Cognitive flexibility

Also known as mental flexibility, this allows individuals to switch between tasks or adjust strategies when situations change. For example, adapting to unexpected changes at work or shifting attention from one task to another when needed.

Planning and organization

This involves the ability to set goals, create a roadmap to achieve them, and effectively manage resources and time. Strong planning skills help individuals break down complex tasks and complete them in a structured, efficient way.

Decision-making

Executive function helps in evaluating options, weighing the pros and cons, and making informed decisions based on logic and experience.

Executive function develops over time, peaking in early adulthood and then gradually declining with age. Enhancing executive function is possible through many of the skills you're learning in this book.

Online Brain Training Games and Apps

Lumosity
Platform: iOS, Android, Web
Lumosity is one of the most popular brain training apps, offering a variety of games that target memory, attention, flexibility, speed of processing, and problem-solving. It customizes challenges based on your performance.

Peak
Platform: iOS, Android
Peak offers over 40 games focused on areas such as memory, language, problem-solving, and emotional control. It includes personalized training plans and detailed performance tracking.

Elevate
Platform: iOS, Android
Elevate features over 35 games designed to improve skills in areas like reading, writing, math, and speaking. It adapts to your skill level and tracks your progress over time.

CogniFit
Platform: iOS, Android, Web
CogniFit provides a range of brain training games and exercises designed to boost cognitive skills like attention, memory, and logical reasoning. It also offers challenges designed for specific age groups.

Brainwell
Platform: iOS, Android
Brainwell includes over 50 games that train various cognitive functions, including memory, attention, and language. It offers personalized brain training programs and allows you to track your progress over time.

Mind Games
Platform: iOS, Android, Web
Mind Games offers a collection of games designed to enhance cognitive abilities such as memory, concentration, and problem-solving. It includes leaderboards to challenge yourself and others.

Fit Brains Trainer
Platform: iOS, Android, Web
Fit Brains Trainer provides games designed to improve memory, concentration, logic, and language. It tracks your performance and suggests personalized training sessions based on your strengths and weaknesses.

NeuroNation
Platform: iOS, Android, Web
NeuroNation offers a variety of brain exercises designed to improve memory, attention, reasoning, and intelligence. The app includes personalized workout plans and tracks progress with detailed reports.

Chess.com
Platform: iOS, Android, Web
Playing chess helps develop strategic thinking, problem-solving, and pattern recognition. Chess.com allows you to play against other users of various skill levels and offers puzzles and lessons to improve your game.

Preserve Your Mental Energy

Everything you do uses mental energy: suppressing distractions, paying attention, processing information, analyzing situations, finding solutions, thinking creatively, make decisions, conduct conversations, access memory, maintain self-control, feel and express empathy, or even meditating.

Even when you aren't aware that your brain is working—while mindlessly perusing TV channels to find entertainment, laughing, or daydreaming, for example—it's tapping into whatever mental energy you've accrued. Your brain is quite literally at the heart of everything you do and sets the agenda for doing anything at all. Here are a few tips for reducing the burden on your brain's energy resources.

Just Say No

Constantly accepting new invitations and opportunities can feel like the right thing to do. But being selective with your time will help to preserve your mental energy. When you spread yourself too thin, you burn out more easily. Constantly taking on new responsibilities can lead to decision fatigue—a condition where your ability to make thoughtful choices deteriorates after making too many decisions. Saying 'no' reduces the number of decisions you need to make, helping conserve mental energy and enabling you to make more deliberate, high-quality choices. It also supports self-care by allowing you to carve out time for rest, reflection, and activities that recharge you, such as exercise, hobbies, or simply relaxing.

Avoid Overthinking

When you overthink, your brain gets stuck in a loop, running simulations of worst-case scenarios or obsessing over past events. The more you ruminate, the more mental resources are depleted, leading to a state of cognitive overload. Your body's stress response is triggered, releasing cortisol, the stress hormone. Elevated cortisol levels can further drain energy, impair concentration, and reduce cognitive function. Chronic overthinking can even interfere with sleep, as the mind remains active, making it difficult to rest and recharge.

Avoid Overworking

As you work longer hours without breaks or rest, mental fatigue sets in. Your brain's ability to concentrate and process information effectively suffers. Chronic overworking negatively impacts the brain's memory systems. Prolonged periods of stress and fatigue can reduce the brain's ability to form and retain new memories, particularly in areas like the hippocampus, responsible for memory consolidation. As a result, you may find it harder to recall information or learn new concepts, even if you've been working on them for hours. Overworking also affects your brain's executive functions, responsible for high-level tasks like decision-making, problem-solving, and planning. Stress and cognitive overload cloud judgment, leading to poor decisions or slower problem-solving abilities. Chronic stress may also shrink areas of the brain associated with memory and emotional regulation. Creativity and innovation thrive when the brain is rested and recharged. Overworking prevents downtime for your brain to engage in restorative processes. This leads to a decrease in creative thinking and the ability to generate new ideas. Mental rest, on the other hand, allows the brain to make connections and think outside the box.

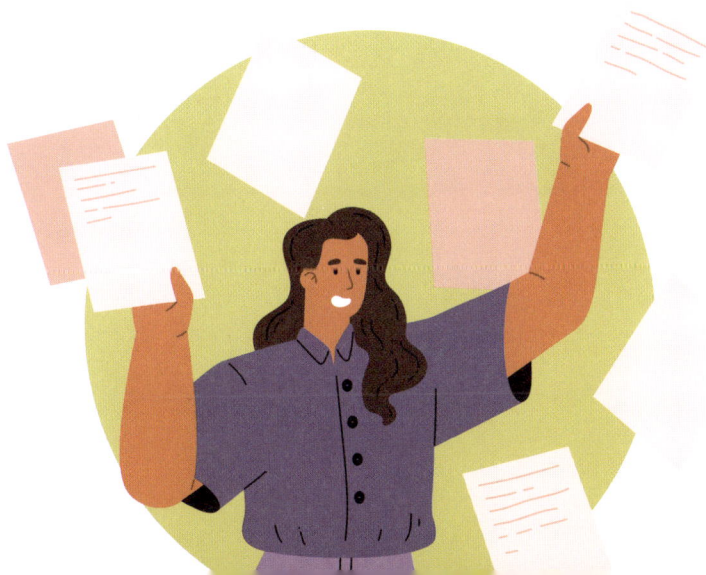

Use this space to reflect upon how doing more and thinking more has decreased your effectiveness, either in work or your personal life.

_____

_____

_____

_____

_____

_____

_____

_____

_____

_____

_____

_____

_____

_____

_____

_____

_____

> **"Daring to set boundaries is about having the courage to love ourselves, even when we risk disappointing others."**
>
> Brené Brown

Now think about how you can rearrange both your schedule and your approach so that you are protecting rather than depleting your mental energy. Use this space to commit to a new approach. Be specific about what you can stop over-doing.

Energy Management

Learning how to work with your natural rhythms can get you in sync with the flow of your day, speed up tasks, maximize productivity and, in turn, save time in your day to do the things that make you happy. The key to becoming more efficient is understanding how your brain works, identifying your flow, and blocking out your time.

Some people may brag about being master multitaskers—perhaps you've even claimed to be one. But multitasking is impossible because the human brain can only focus on one thing at time. What you're experiencing when you claim to be multitasking is your brain rapidly switching from one area of focus to another. This wastes valuable brain power and proves to be an inefficient way to function.

In fact, multitasking trains your brain to behave poorly. Each task, regardless of how small, that you "complete" (like responding to a text message) releases dopamine, the reward hormone, in your brain. This surge of "happiness" trains your brain to jump from small task to small task just to receive more dopamine. You should fight this tendency and instead focus efficiently on a single task for the even greater reward of freeing up the time that you would have otherwise wasted while multitasking.

What you consider to be multitasking is harming you in the following ways:

◊   Creates mental exhaustion so you lose valuable energy that could be used on the things you enjoy

◊   Lowers the quality of your work and makes you more inefficient

◊   Increases stress levels by boosting production of the stress hormone cortisol

◊   Reduces productivity by 40 percent.

Match Your Schedule to Your Internal Clock

Most people perform better during a certain time of day. Some are fired up and ready to work early in the morning; for others, their best work occurs later in the day. Your peak focus time is impacted by your natural circadian rhythm. Most people focus the best around 11:00 am or closer to 4 pm If you're an early bird, it could be much earlier than 11:00 am. If you're not an early riser, you might not hit your stride until mid-afternoon.

Identify Your Energy Levels

To take full advantage of your peak energy levels you need to know when they occur. This requires mindful observation over a period of time to notice when you feel most alert and energized versus when you experience energy dips.

Typically, energy peaks in the morning hours, shortly after waking up, then most often lulls after lunch, in the early afternoon. However, this can vary significantly from person to person, influenced by lifestyle, sleep habits, and even genetics.

To gather accurate information on your energy levels, monitor and record them in a diary for a few weeks. Note the times of day when you feel and act most alert and productive and those when you feel fatigued and find it harder to focus. Look for patterns and consider how your current schedule aligns—or doesn't—with these energy levels.

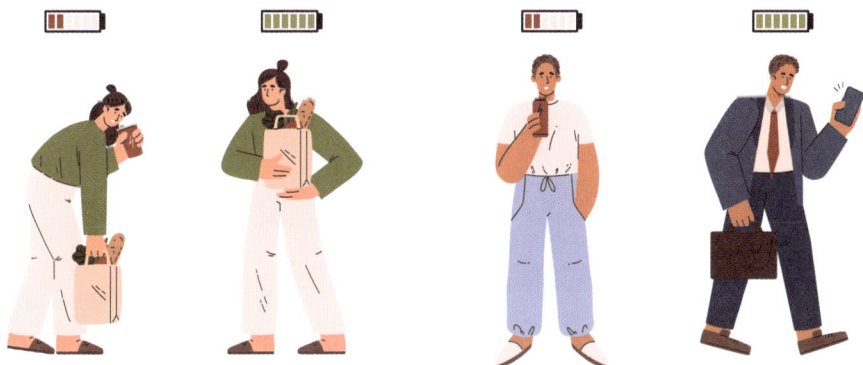

Align Your Energy

It's important to know your body's rhythm and identify those times of the day when your brain is most alert. Once you know your peak hours, structure your day around them, focusing on activities that require the most effort and creativity for your peak hours .

Once you align how you work with how your body/brain functions, you'll both preserve energy and be much more efficient.

Match Tasks to Energy Levels

Once you've identified your energy patterns, you can take advantage of your natural rhythm. High-energy periods are ideal for the most demanding or challenging tasks that require deep focus or creative thinking. Conversely, low-energy periods are better suited for administrative tasks, meetings, emails, or activities that require less cognitive effort. For example, if you're a morning person, dedicate your early hours to strategic planning or creative projects and save emails or routine check-ins for the post-lunch slump.

Adapting your routine to maximize your energy levels may require experimentation and adjustment. Start by shifting your most important tasks to your identified peak times, then monitor how doing so affects your productivity and overall energy throughout the day.

You might also find it helpful to experiment with different types of breaks to see which ones rejuvenate your low-energy periods. Try alternating activities, such as taking short brisk walks, meditating, or taking a brief nap. You can also monitor exercise and how it affects energy levels, and if you want to take it a step further, monitor when and what you eat and how it affects your energy levels.

This process may seem tedious at first, but it might reveal the need for changes in your sleep habits, exercise routine, or diet—all of which play critical roles in energy management and overall circadian health. Minor adjustments in these areas can lead to improvements in how you feel and perform each day.

"Energy is the essence of life. Every day you decide how you're going to use it by knowing what you want and what it takes to reach that goal, and by maintaining focus."

Oprah Winfrey

☐ **High Energy** ☐ **Medium Energy** ☐ **Low Energy**

	1am	2am	3am	4am	5am	6am	7am	8am	9am	10am	11am
MONDAY											
TUESDAY											
WEDNEDAY											
THURSDAY											
FRIDAY											
SATURDAY											
SUNDAY											

12am	1am	2am	3am	4am	5am	6am	7am	8am	9am	10am	11am	12am

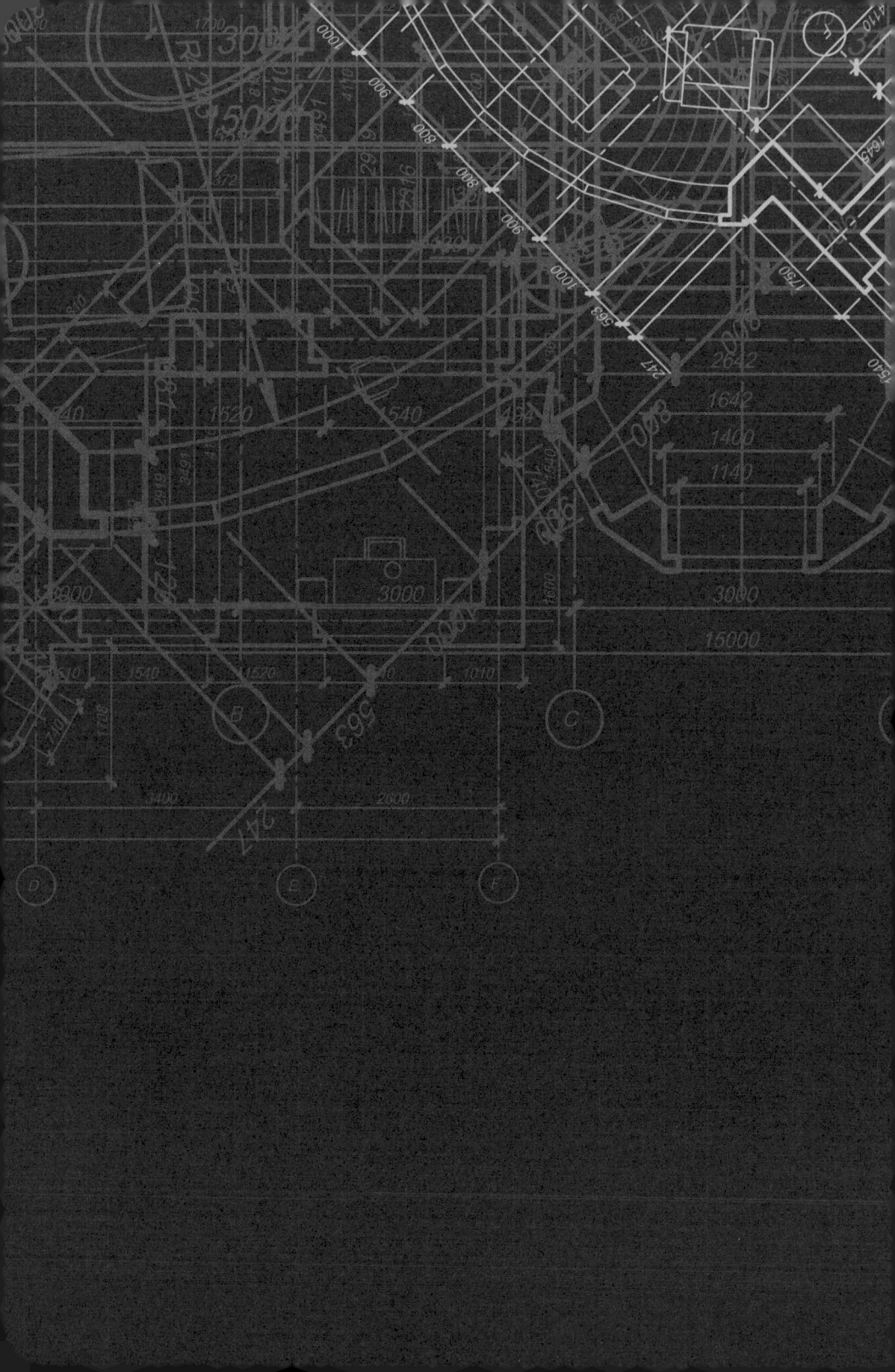

Mindfulness and Meditation

A

What is Mindfulness?

Mindfulness is the practice of focusing your attention on the present moment, with an attitude of openness, curiosity, and non-judgment. It involves paying full attention to your thoughts, emotions, physical sensations, and the environment around you, without becoming overwhelmed by them or reacting impulsively. The essence of mindfulness is cultivating awareness and acceptance, allowing you to experience each moment as it is, without being influenced by past experiences or future worries.

At its core, mindfulness involves awareness and acceptance. Awareness refers to being fully engaged in the present moment, while acceptance means observing your experiences without judgment, avoiding the urge to label them as 'good' or 'bad.' It's about noticing what's happening inside and around you, without getting caught up in any emotional reaction. This might involve paying attention to the breath, bodily sensations, or the surrounding environment, as well as acknowledging your thoughts and emotions with curiosity instead of criticism.

Mindfulness can be practiced formally, through techniques such as meditation, or informally, by integrating mindful awareness into daily activities such as eating, walking, or even listening.

Mindfulness helps reduce stress and anxiety. When we are stressed or anxious, we often find ourselves ruminating about past events or worrying about the future, which can cause our stress levels to skyrocket. Mindfulness encourages us to focus on the present, which can disrupt these negative thought patterns. By practicing mindfulness, we can break the cycle of rumination, lower our levels of cortisol (the body's stress hormone), and cultivate a more relaxed state of mind.

Numerous studies show that mindfulness meditation can help reduce the physiological effects of stress. It has been shown to help individuals manage anxiety disorders, such as generalized anxiety disorder (GAD) and social anxiety disorder, by fostering a sense of calm and control over one's thoughts.

Mindfulness helps us become more aware of our emotions, allowing us to respond to feelings in a healthier way. It enhances emotional regulation by encouraging us to to observe their emotions without immediately reacting to them. This awareness allows us to identify negative emotions early, enabling us to choose a more measured response rather than impulsively reacting with frustration, anger, or sadness.

Mindfulness also encourages self-compassion, which helps us to break patterns of self-criticism and improves overall emotional resilience. By accepting emotions as part of the human experience, we learn not to suppress them or let them control us. This emotional awareness can lead to greater emotional intelligence and the ability to relate more effectively to others.

Mindfulness practices, particularly meditation, train the brain to focus on a single point of attention. Over time, this increases your ability to concentrate and improves your working memory. By learning to focus on the present moment, mindfulness helps you filter out distractions and remain engaged in tasks, which can boost productivity and overall cognitive performance.

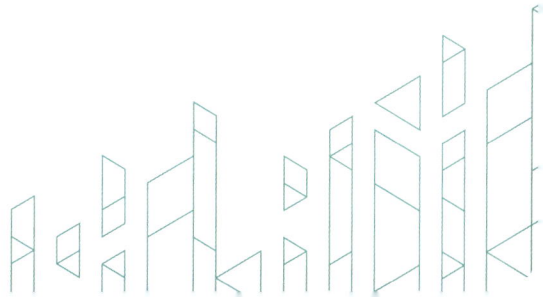

Many studies demonstrate that mindfulness can increase gray matter in areas of the brain related to memory, decision-making, and self-control. People who practice mindfulness regularly tend to show greater cognitive flexibility and improved attention span. This can be especially beneficial in situations where sustained focus is required, such as studying, working, or solving complex problems.

Mindfulness also enhances social skills by improving your ability to listen attentively and respond with empathy. Being present and fully engaged in a conversation allows for deeper connections and fosters more meaningful relationships. It helps you tune into the emotions of others without judgment, improving both personal and professional relationships. In a study of couples, mindfulness training has been shown to lead to more effective communication and greater emotional intimacy. By being present with your partner—listening without distraction and responding with care—mindfulness can improve the quality of relationships.

Mindfulness doesn't just benefit mental well-being—it has a positive impact on physical health as well. Research suggests that mindfulness practices can reduce blood pressure, reduce chronic pain, improve sleep quality, and boost immune system functioning. By lowering stress levels and fostering a sense of calm, mindfulness has the potential to prevent or mitigate the physical symptoms that arise from chronic stress, such as headaches, muscle tension, and digestive issues.

Mindfulness fosters a sense of balance and presence, encouraging people to prioritize self-care, take breaks when needed, and be kinder to themselves. This balanced approach is crucial for avoiding burnout in our fast-paced, always-connected world. By integrating mindfulness into daily life, we are reminded to slow down, appreciate the present, and avoid getting lost in the pressures and demands of modern life.

In a world filled with constant distractions and demands, mindfulness offers a way to reconnect with the present, foster inner peace, and improve resilience. Whether through meditation or simply practicing mindful awareness in everyday activities, integrating mindfulness into your life can lead to a deeper sense of well-being and a more balanced, fulfilling life.

Basic Mindfulness Exercise

This simple exercise can be done anytime and anywhere to bring you firmly into the experience of your present moment. By recognizing your five senses, which are working all the time even if you don't notice them, you acknowledge your present experience. It is this acknowledgment that brings your consciousness back to here and now.

Ask yourself the following questions and respond in your mind. Or if you're somewhere private, you can say your answers out loud.

Sound   What do I hear?

_____

Sight   What do I see?

_____

Smell   What do I smell?

_____

Taste   What do I taste

_____

Touch   What do I feel?

_____

Do this exercise daily. If you find yourself feeling stuck in the past or the future, repeat this exercise numerous times a day until staying in the moment becomes a habit.

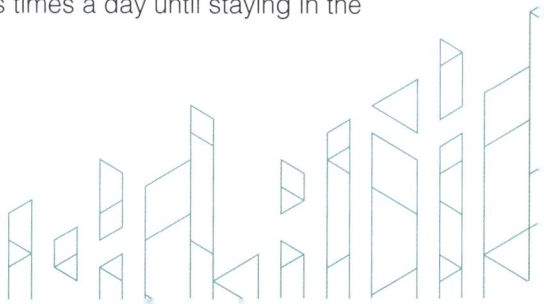

Mindfulness in Nature

Try this exercise in a local park, woodland, nature reserve or garden, if you have access to these.

1. Find a green space. When you get there, stop for a moment and take a deep breath. Start exploring slowly. Try not to focus on getting somewhere in particular. Really focus on any movement you make. If you're walking, notice which part of your foot touches the ground first, and feel the transfer of weight through your foot.

2. Notice the ground underneath you. Is it grass or earth? Does the ground feel soft? What colors can you see?

3. Think about the rest of your body. How are you holding your arms? Does the air on your face feel cold or warm?

4. Listen to the sounds around you. Can you hear birdsong, or wind, rustling through the leaves?

If you can't go to a green space, you can try opening your window and noticing what's around you. Notice any clouds in the sky, or trees and plants you can see. Can you feel rain, wind or sun on your skin?

You could try looking after a plant. Spend time focusing on its scent, shape, and texture. You could try touching some of the leaves or soil and focusing on how it feels.

10 Ways To Reconnect Your Mind, Body, and Spirit

1. Turn off all electronics during meals

2. Practice gratitude

3. Do a body scan and check in with how you are feeling

4. Stop and ask your heart how it is feeling

5. Stop and check in with your five senses

6. Take a deep breath or three

7. Put down your fork in between each bite; savor each one

8. Listen fully and with intention

9. Walk barefoot on the grass, beach, or soil

10. Stop and look around; notice where you can find the beauty in the everyday

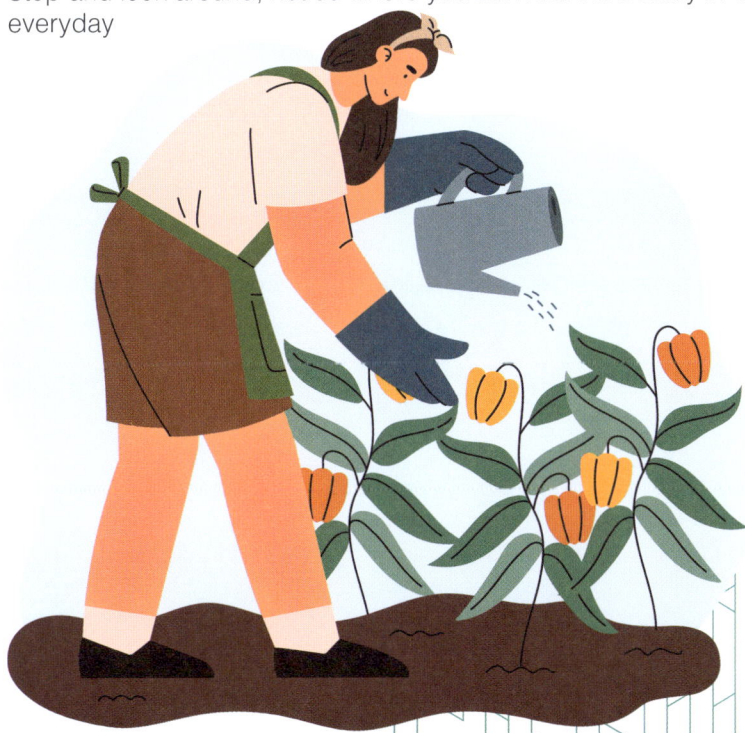

Why Meditate?

While meditation is often associated with stress-reduction, it can also be great for mental focus. Research has shown that regular meditation practice can have both short-term and long-term effects on brain health and performance.

Meditation improves your ability to focus and pay attention. Mindfulness meditation trains the mind to maintain sustained attention on a single task or thought while reducing distractions. This enhanced focus is linked to changes in the prefrontal cortex, the brain region responsible for decision-making, problem-solving, and goal-setting. Studies have shown that meditators tend to perform better on tasks requiring concentration and working memory.

Because chronic stress can impair memory and reduce cognitive flexibility, meditation's role in reducing the body's stress response and lowering levels of cortisol can help your brain to remain open and responsive. By fostering a calm, present state of mind, meditation helps individuals process information more clearly and make decisions with greater ease. Studies using brain imaging techniques have demonstrated that long-term meditators show increased gray matter density in areas related to learning, memory, and emotional regulation, such as the hippocampus and anterior cingulate cortex. These changes suggest that regular meditation not only improves cognitive performance but may also protect against age-related cognitive decline.

For the uninitiated, meditating may look easy, and in fact appear as though you are just 'sitting there doing nothing' except breathing. While it can be simple, there's more to it. It takes time and practice to achieve a meditative state. Trying the techniques on the following pages on a sustained basis will help you get there.

"Meditation is like a gym in which you develop the powerful mental muscles of calm and insight."

Ajahn Brahm

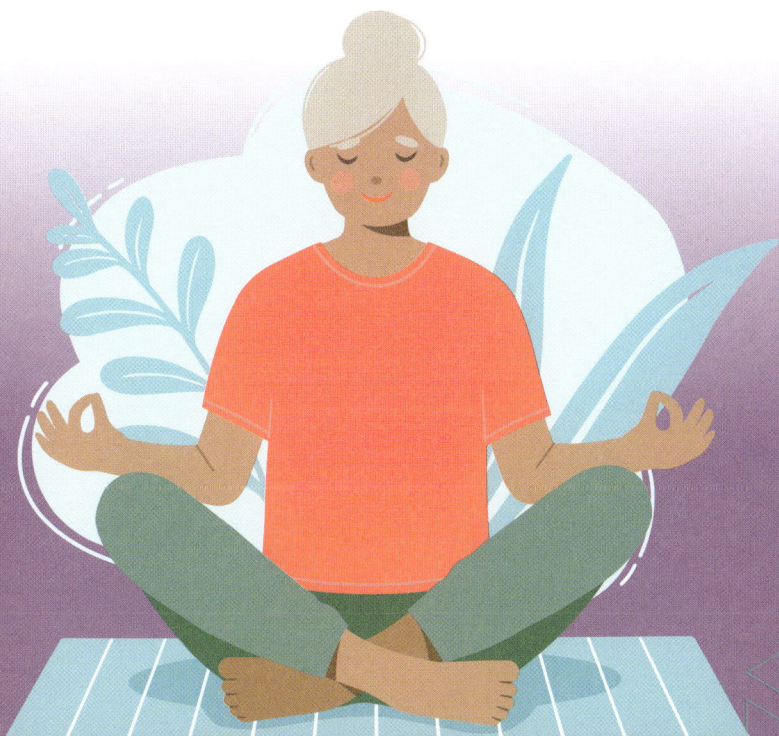

Meditation Basics

Chances are, you can find a mediation group or class near you or online. Often it helps to have a mentor or teacher who can help you begin to feel comfortable with the process of meditation. But you can also work on it on your own.

1. Find a secluded spot where you can sit without interruption. You can participate in this practice in silence, or you can choose to play some calming music. If you choose to listen to music, choose something instrumental or ambient. You can find free meditation playlists easily online or you can make your own.

2. Settle in so that you feel as comfortable as possible. Close your eyes and begin to breathe slowly, deeply, and intentionally. Breathe in through your nose and out of your mouth. Feel the breath enter your lungs. If you are breathing deeply while relaxed, you will feel your belly rise and fall with your breath.

3. Follow or track your breath. In. Out. Follow the air as it makes its way through your nose, all the way down into your lungs and belly, and then as it travels back upward to exit your body out of your mouth. Keep breathing and tracking your breath slowly and rhythmically. If a thought or feeling pops up that distracts you from focusing on your breath, acknowledge the thought without judgment. Then release it. This can be difficult to do. Imagine yourself as a passive observer of your thoughts who is not directly connected to them. Give the thought a moment of attention. Then let it go. Bring your attention back to your breath.

> ## "Feelings come and go like clouds in a windy sky. Conscious breathing is my anchor."
>
> Thich Nhat Hanh

4. You are meditating and focusing on following your breath. You begin to feel peaceful, calm, and centered. Suddenly you think about what you need to make for dinner. You step back in your mind's eye to observe the thought. Your internal observer thinks, "Hmm, I just thought about what I need to make for dinner. That is what was present in my mind. I choose to release that thought. All I have to do right now to be exactly where I am focusing on my breath." And then you refocus on your breath and continue to meditate.

Note: Having thoughts during meditation is completely normal. Instead of viewing the time spent acknowledging your thoughts as a setback, shift your perspective. Every thought that pops up and that you acknowledge is something new you have learned about your internal programming. The more you learn about yourself, the better you can be.

Continue to repeat steps 3 and 4. You can practice for five minutes, thirty minutes, or even an hour. There is no set amount of time to devote to your practice. Just keep practicing for optimum results!

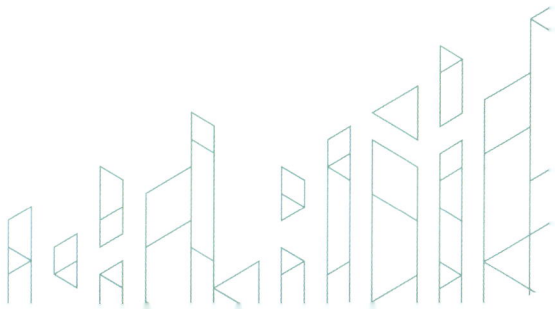

Body Scan Meditation

The body scan helps to increase body awareness and promote relaxation, reducing physical and mental tension.

Find a comfortable lying position, either on your back with your arms by your sides or sitting with a relaxed posture.

Close your eyes and take a few deep breaths to relax.

Begin by bringing your attention to your toes. Notice any sensations in your feet—whether they are warm, cool, tense, or relaxed.

Slowly move your attention upward through your body. Gradually scan each part of your body, from your toes to your head, paying attention to any tension, discomfort, or areas of relaxation.

If you notice tension, simply observe it without judgment. Breathe into the area and imagine releasing the tension as you exhale.

Continue scanning and breathing through your entire body. Take your time to really connect with how your body feels in each area.

After you've scanned your whole body, take a few deep breaths and relax fully into the present moment before ending the practice.

> "When meditation is mastered, the mind is unwavering like the flame of a candle in a windless place."
>
> The Bhagavad Gita

Loving-Kindness Meditation

The Loving-Kindess meditation cultivates compassion, empathy, and a sense of connectedness with others, while also improving your own emotional well-being.

Sit in a comfortable, upright position and close your eyes.

Take a few deep breaths to center yourself.

Begin by silently repeating the following phrases, directing them toward yourself:

◊   "May I be happy."   ◊   "May I be safe."

◊   "May I be healthy."   ◊   "May I live with ease."

After several rounds of sending kindness to yourself, gradually expand the practice. Recall someone you care about and repeat the same phrases for them:

◊   "May you be happy."   ◊   "May you be safe."

◊   "May you be healthy."   ◊   "May you live with ease."

Next, extend these wishes to others—perhaps a neutral person, someone you have difficulty with, or even all beings everywhere.

Continue to repeat these phrases, allowing the feelings of kindness to expand outward.

When you feel ready, close the practice by returning to your own well-being and gratitude.

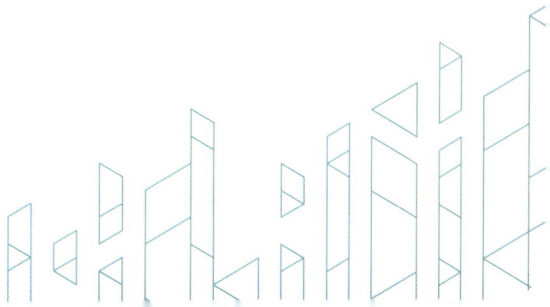

Tense and Release

Our bodies are well equipped to manage healthy levels of daily stress. However, when we experience heightened levels of stress and anxiety, our brain thinks we are in danger. This sends our body into fight-or-flight mode, causing our muscles to tighten. Yet, when no real threat is present, this constant muscle tension can lead to chronic pain, illness, and decreased emotional well-being. By deliberately tensing, then relaxing, each muscle group in a particular order, you can reduce muscle tension and decrease stress and anxiety.

1. Find a relaxing and comfortable space. You can do this exercise while lying down on a soft surface or sitting in a comfortable chair. Be sure to uncross your arms, legs, and ankles.

2. Begin by taking three balloon breaths (see page 149) while allowing your body to fall into a relaxed state.

3. Bring your awareness to your toes. Take a deep balloon breath in and tense and flex your toes for five to ten seconds. Be sure to notice how this tension feels in your body.

4. Take a deep balloon breath out as you immediately release the tension in your toes. This should be a sudden release rather than gradual.

5. Take about fifteen seconds to relax and regroup. Bring your awareness to your body, with specific attention to your toes. How do they feel now compared to when you had them tensed?

6. Repeat steps 2 to 5 for each of the following muscle groups in this order:

Feet	Arms (lower and bicep)
Bottom half of legs	Shoulders
Thighs	Neck
Buttocks	Jaw
Stomach	Face
Back (lower, middle, shoulder blade area)	Lips/smile, nose, eyes
Hands	Forehead

7. Relax for twenty seconds, then tense your entire body and release for ten seconds.

8. Take some time to stretch and breathe. Count backward from ten to slowly bring yourself back to the present moment. Take your time getting up as you may feel a bit lightheaded.

What did you notice after doing this exercise?

_____

_____

_____

_____

_____

_____

_____

_____

_____

_____

_____

_____

_____

_____

Mountain Meditation

Close your eyes and bring to mind a tall, steady mountain. See its solid base, rooted deep into the earth, and its peak rising high into the sky. Imagine yourself becoming this mountain—strong, unmoving, and calm. Feel your body sitting tall, spine straight, grounded like the base of the mountain.

Notice how the mountain endures all seasons: the warmth of the sun, the chill of snow, the rush of storms, and the quiet of clear skies. No matter what passes across its surface, the mountain remains steady at its core. Breathe deeply, drawing in stability with every inhale, and releasing tension with every exhale.

Allow yourself to embody the strength, patience, and stillness of this mountain. As thoughts come and go, see them as passing clouds—temporary, drifting, and harmless. Rest in the quiet presence of your mountain nature, unshaken, deeply at peace.

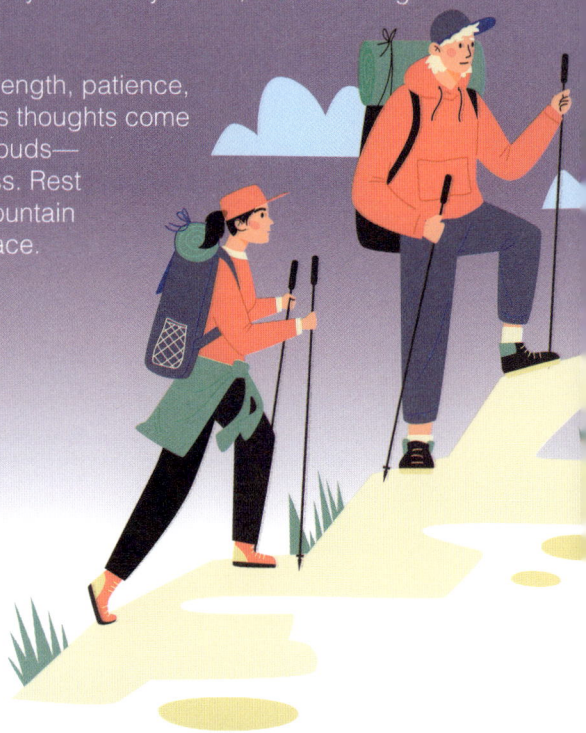

Breathwork

Breathwork refers to breathing practices believed to be therapeutic. You can engage in these practices for anywhere from a few minutes to an hour. You can time breathing in and out, holding your breath, or both. Breathwork helps people get to the mental state they are seeking when meditating, but much faster. In fact, breathwork can help detach you from your thoughts entirely, which can allow healing and relaxation to occur at a swift pace.

Breathwork has numerous benefits, including:

◊   Reducing stress   ◊   Improving the immune system

◊   Lowering blood pressure   ◊   Increasing joy

◊   Releasing trauma   ◊   Processing emotions.

You can learn to practice breathwork in a variety of ways. Much like yoga and meditation, you can choose to find a breathwork teacher or attend a class or workshop. You can also find courses and guided breathwork sessions online. There are apps that you can download that help you create your own breathwork routine. You can research the practice online and create your own breathwork practice.

Breathwork is beneficial for sleep because it allows you to release the stressors of the day. It can bring you to a centered and present place, which helps to reduce depression and anxiety. It can also bring you to a clear-headed space, which is an ideal mindset for restful sleep.
When you begin your practice, listen to your body. Everyone has a different experience with breathwork. For some it is mild and for others it can be a total mind-body experience. When you first start your breathwork journey, it is important to practice in a safe place while lying down. This is vital because many people get light-headed or experience tingling or chills when they begin their practice. If, at any time, breathwork feels straining on the body or mind, take a break.

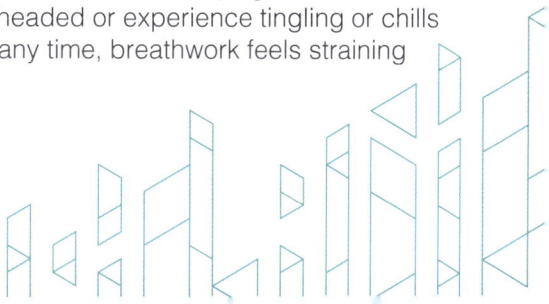

Getting Started

To begin your breathwork practice, start by learning to breathe deeply and to use your breath for relaxation. This is a wonderful practice in the evening to prepare for sleep.

Find a quiet spot. You can choose to partake in this practice in silence or you can play music. This can be any relaxing music of your choice.

Lie down somewhere comfortable where you can fully stretch out. This can be on a couch, on your bed, or on a mat.

Place your hands lightly on top of your belly.

Breathe in deeply through your nose for a count of 4. Bring the breath down into the belly. Watch your belly rise and feel it fill up with air.

Exhale out of your mouth for a count of 8. Continue to do this for ten minutes.

At the end of the practice, take note of how you feel. Are your limbs more relaxed? Do you feel more present and aware? Does your mind feel clear? Did you release some stress in your body and mind? Use the space below to reflect.

_____

_____

_____

_____

_____

_____

_____

Balloon Breathing

As we get older, the way in which we breathe tends to change. We experience more life stessors and triggers, and as a result, our bodies can become more dysregulated. We tend to do more of what's called 'shoulder shrug breathing.' When we take a breath in, our chest and shoulders lift upward; when we exhale, our shoulders and chest fall back down. While it may seem like a quicker way to get a breath, this way of breathing drastically limits the amount of air we can take into our lungs. Yet, these short shoulder-shrug breaths do serve a distinct purpose. In fight-or-flight mode, shorter breaths allow oxygen to get into our lungs in the fastest way possible. They increase our heart rate, make our blood pump faster, and increase the production of the stress hormone cortisol—all vital body responses when we are facing a threat. The problem is that most of us use shoulder-shrug breathing when we are not facing a real threat of danger. This tricks our body into responding as if we were in danger, often putting us at higher risk for anxiety and/or a panic attack.

If you look at babies and animals, you will notice that when they breathe, their stomachs move up and down, not their chests. This is proper breathing technique. When we take a breath in, our stomachs should rise with air; when we exhale, our stomachs should go down. We can get deeper, slower, more controlled breaths. Our chest and shoulders, when engaged in proper breathing technique, shouldn't really move at all! This "balloon breathing" exercise teaches proper breathing technique to help regulate our bodies and reduce stress and anxiety.

Now, pick your favorite color balloon. Imagine this balloon in your belly. While standing in front of the mirror again:

1. Take a deep breath in for five seconds while visualizing your balloon filling up with air.

2. Hold for five seconds.

3. Exhale to a count of five while visualizing your balloon deflating in your belly.

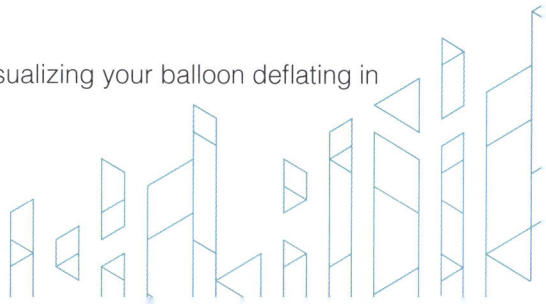

Which body parts moved this time for you? Did you notice how your breathing was deeper and slower, allowing for calmer breaths?

Try practicing this exercise three times a day while in a relatively relaxed state of mind. Your ability to be mindful of your breath will be significantly better when you are not distracted by stress and worry.

After a week or so of practicing this exercise, do you notice anything different about your breathing or your response in stressful situations?

_____

_____

_____

_____

_____

_____

_____

_____

_____

_____

_____

_____

Count and Breathe Yourself to Sleep

This controlled breathing exercise is perfect for those nights when you lie down, close your eyes, and cannot fall asleep. Instead of counting sheep, try counting your breath. This commonly recommended 4-7-8 breath practice allows your body to slow down, relaxes the pace of your heart, and helps release anxiety.

1. In your bed with the lights off, comfortably lie on your back. You can keep the pillow under your head for this exercise because, ideally, you will drift off to sleep before you complete it!

2. Place your hands on your belly or rest your arms gently to your sides. Relax your arms and legs.

3. With your eyes closed, breathe in through your nose for the count of 4.

4. Visualize this breath making its way all the way down to your belly.

5. Gently hold this breath for the count of 7.

6. Release this breath for the count of 8.

Repeat this cycle for ten minutes or until you fall asleep. If you are not asleep or ready for sleep at the end of the ten minutes, you can repeat this practice again.

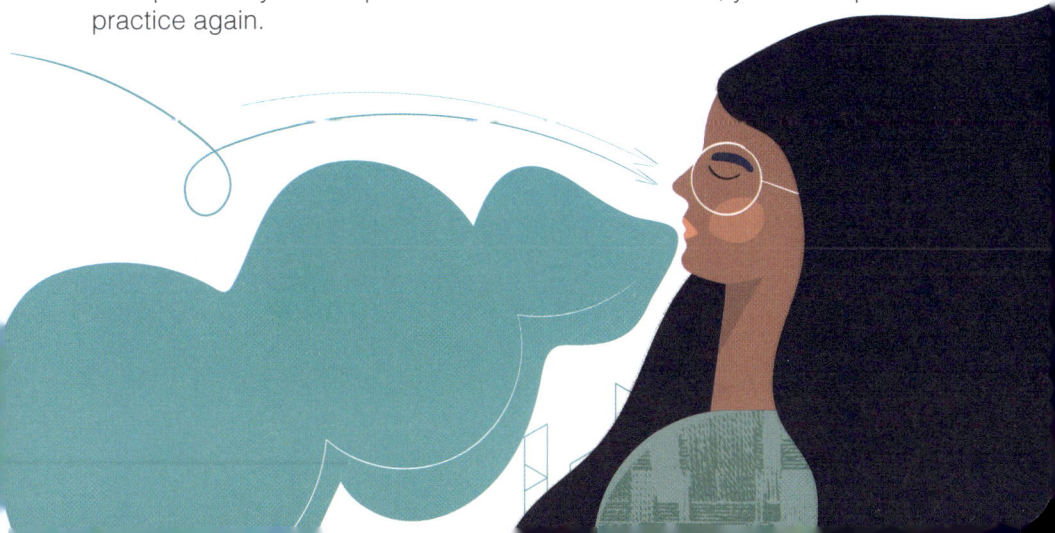

Journaling

While it may seem very old-school and analog, journaling is among the best tools for enhancing your mental clarity. When you write down your thoughts and summarize information, you're reinforcing your memory. The act of organizing thoughts on paper can improve your retention and recall because your brain is actively processing. When you journal, you're often reflecting on events or concepts, helping to commit information to your long-term memory.

Journaling helps clear mental clutter by allowing you to process emotions, thoughts, and stressors. By writing out your concerns or ideas, you free up mental space, making it easier to focus and think critically. This process of decluttering the mind can lead to improved problem-solving and clearer thinking in other areas of life. Regular journaling engages the brain in a deep focus state, which can translate into improved attention span over time.

By providing a safe space for expressing emotions, journaling can improve emotional regulation, essential for mental sharpness because it prevents mental fatigue and distraction caused by unmanaged emotions. It can also help with creativity and problem solving.

You can also engage in goal setting, planning, and organization. The process of reflecting on your day or setting intentions for the future encourages the use of executive functions such as decision-making, prioritizing tasks, and managing time effectively.

Morning Pages

Setting aside five minutes each morning to connect with yourself is one of the most important things you can do to set yourself up for a good day. If you don't have five minutes in the morning to write, set your alarm five minutes earlier than normal. These extra five minutes can have a massive impact on the rest of your day if you use them correctly.

If you make it a daily habit, the following exercise can reduce anxiety, increase joy, and help you focus. How does it work? Your 'morning pages' let you acknowledge and let go of pain points. They give you clear, achievable objectives for the day, help set your mood, and shift you to a space of gratitude, imagination, and hope. This exercise is so effective it can feel like you took a magic mood-boosting pill. Use the following pages to begin a practice that you can continue in a journal of your choosing. Each page should include following elements.

A Structure for Morning Pages

Thoughts - Leave space here to write freely. Put anything and everything you're thinking about in this section. Get it out of your head and on to the page. This helps you clear space for the thoughts that you want to consciously put into your mind.

To Be Completed - Don't exceed six goals for the day, but these goals should be achievable within a single day. Use this section to get a clear view of your objectives for the day and celebrate each time you check something off the list.

Intention - Write down who you want to show up as today.

Gratitude - Write down three very specific things you're grateful for.

Dreams - Write exactly what you're hoping for, wishing for, or manifesting for your future.

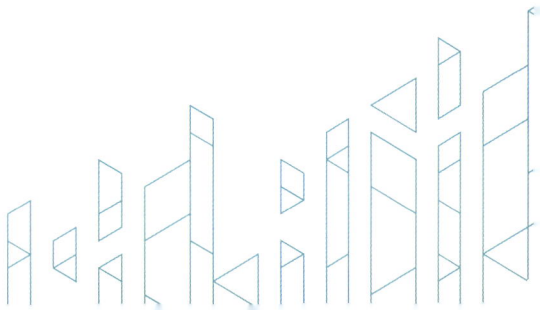

Morning Page

DAY OF THE WEEK

THOUGHTS

TO BE COMPLETED

- [ ]
- [ ]
- [ ]
- [ ]
- [ ]
- [ ]

INTENTION

GRATITUDE

1.
2.
3.

DREAMS

1.
2.
3.

Morning Page

DAY OF THE WEEK

THOUGHTS

TO BE COMPLETED

- [ ]
- [ ]
- [ ]
- [ ]
- [ ]
- [ ]

INTENTION

GRATITUDE

1.
2.
3.

DREAMS

1.
2.
3.

Morning Page

DAY OF THE WEEK

THOUGHTS

TO BE COMPLETED

- [ ]
- [ ]
- [ ]
- [ ]
- [ ]
- [ ]

INTENTION

GRATITUDE

1.
2.
3.

DREAMS

1.
2.
3.

Morning Page

DAY OF THE WEEK

THOUGHTS

TO BE COMPLETED

- [ ]
- [ ]
- [ ]
- [ ]
- [ ]
- [ ]

INTENTION

GRATITUDE

1.
2.
3.

DREAMS

1.
2.
3.

Morning Page

DAY OF THE WEEK

THOUGHTS

TO BE COMPLETED

- [ ]
- [ ]
- [ ]
- [ ]
- [ ]
- [ ]

INTENTION

GRATITUDE

1.
2.
3.

DREAMS

1.
2.
3.

Morning Page

DAY OF THE WEEK

THOUGHTS

TO BE COMPLETED

- [ ]
- [ ]
- [ ]
- [ ]
- [ ]
- [ ]

INTENTION

GRATITUDE

1.
2.
3.

DREAMS

1.
2.
3.

Morning Page

DAY OF THE WEEK

THOUGHTS

TO BE COMPLETED

- [ ]
- [ ]
- [ ]
- [ ]
- [ ]
- [ ]

INTENTION

GRATITUDE

1.
2.
3.

DREAMS

1.
2.
3.

Morning Page

DAY OF THE WEEK

THOUGHTS

TO BE COMPLETED

- [ ]
- [ ]
- [ ]
- [ ]
- [ ]
- [ ]

INTENTION

GRATITUDE

1.
2.
3.

DREAMS

1.
2.
3.

Jumpstart Your Journaling

Journaling can sharpen cognitive functions such as memory and comprehension by organizing your thoughts coherently. Tracking progress, gratitude, or daily accomplishments boosts motivation and positivity, which are key to maintaining mental resilience.

Setting aside time to journal can become a mindfulness practice, grounding you in the present moment and improving focus. Over time, this habit strengthens your ability to cope with life's challenges, improve relationships, and cultivate gratitude.

In short, journaling offers a reflective space to manage stress, boost mental clarity, and nurture emotional health. Making journaling part of your routine is an investment in your well-being that pays lasting dividends.

On those days when you are at a loss for what to journal about use the prompts on the following pages to get you started.

> "Journaling is an offshoot of meditation— a type of introspection where a record of events is welcome. It doesn't have to mean the record is permanent. In fact, it's probably better as ephemeral— permanently locked behind a password. But the fact that it exists is a comfort in itself."
>
> C.J. Chilvers

I am my most authentic self when I do the following things:

What do I have in common with the people who cause me the most stress in my life?

What are the values I hold most dear?

What would I do if I had an extra hour every day?

_____

_____

_____

_____

_____

_____

_____

_____

_____

_____

_____

_____

_____

_____

_____

_____

_____

_____

_____

_____

_____

What does success mean to me?

What is my most cherished possession? What does it say about me that I chose this?

_____

_____

_____

_____

_____

_____

_____

_____

_____

_____

_____

_____

_____

_____

_____

_____

_____

_____

_____

_____

What truth do I need to confront?

When was the last time I changed my mind about something? How did that happen? Am I too rigid in my thinking? If so, how can I change that?

If I could go back and talk to my previous self at any age, what time would I go to and what would I say?

_____

_____

_____

_____

_____

_____

_____

_____

_____

_____

_____

_____

_____

_____

_____

_____

_____

_____

_____

_____

What parts of my personality am I holding back on? How could I free them so I feel more complete as a person?

_____

_____

_____

_____

_____

_____

_____

_____

_____

_____

_____

_____

_____

_____

_____

_____

_____

_____

_____

_____

_____

_____

What's one thing I can let go of today, mentally or emotionally?

Brain Games for Mental Stimulation

Brain Games

Just as physical exercise strengthens muscles and supports cardiovascular health, mental stimulation helps build and preserve the brain's neural networks, fostering cognitive resilience well into old age. Engaging in mentally challenging activities including puzzles, strategy games, and memory exercises promotes neuroplasticity, which helps counteract age-related cognitive decline and reduces the risk of neurodegenerative diseases such as Alzheimer's and other forms of dementia.

Research shows that people who regularly engage in brain-stimulating games and activities tend to maintain better memory, attention, and problem-solving skills. These cognitive benefits contribute to greater independence and quality of life as we age. While the games included on the following pages are done solor, you can also find mentally stimulating games also encourage social interaction.

Beyond brain health, mental engagement has been linked to lower stress levels, better mood regulation, and improved sleep—all of which influence longevity. Challenging the mind keeps it resilient to the physical and emotional stresses that can accelerate aging.

Incorporating brain games into daily routines is a fun, accessible way to keep your mind sharp. Whether it's crossword puzzles, Sudoku, memory card games, or even learning a new language or musical instrument, these activities serve as a workout for your brain, helping to preserve mental acuity and supporting a longer, vibrant life. Use the games on the following pages as a jumping off point for finding out what kind of mentally stimulating games work for you.

Maze 1

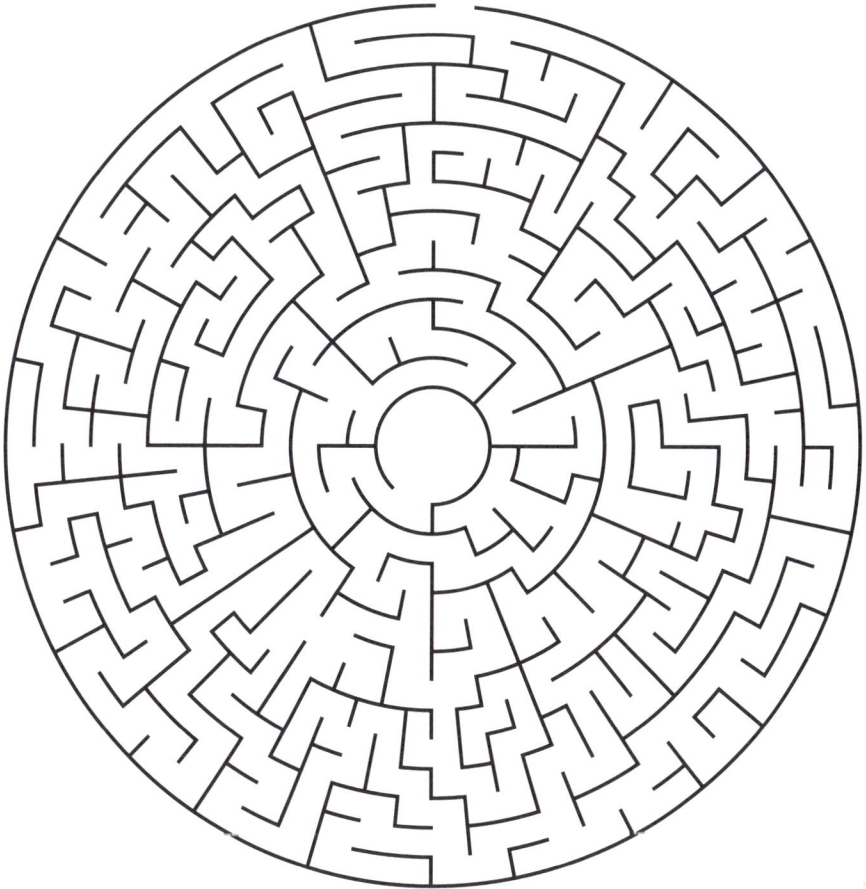
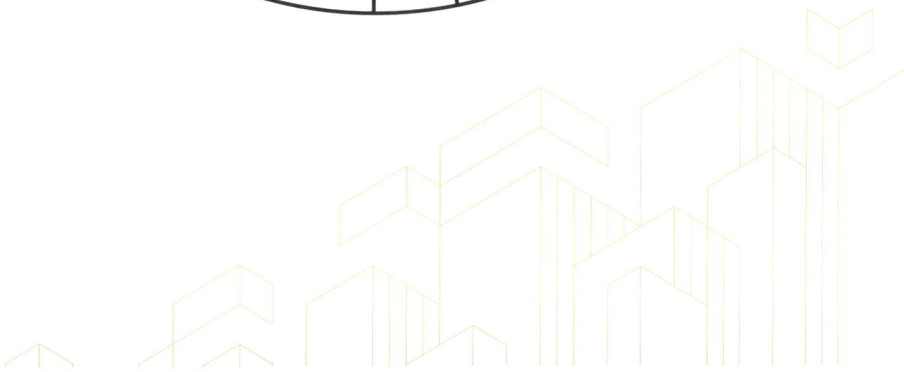

Maze 2

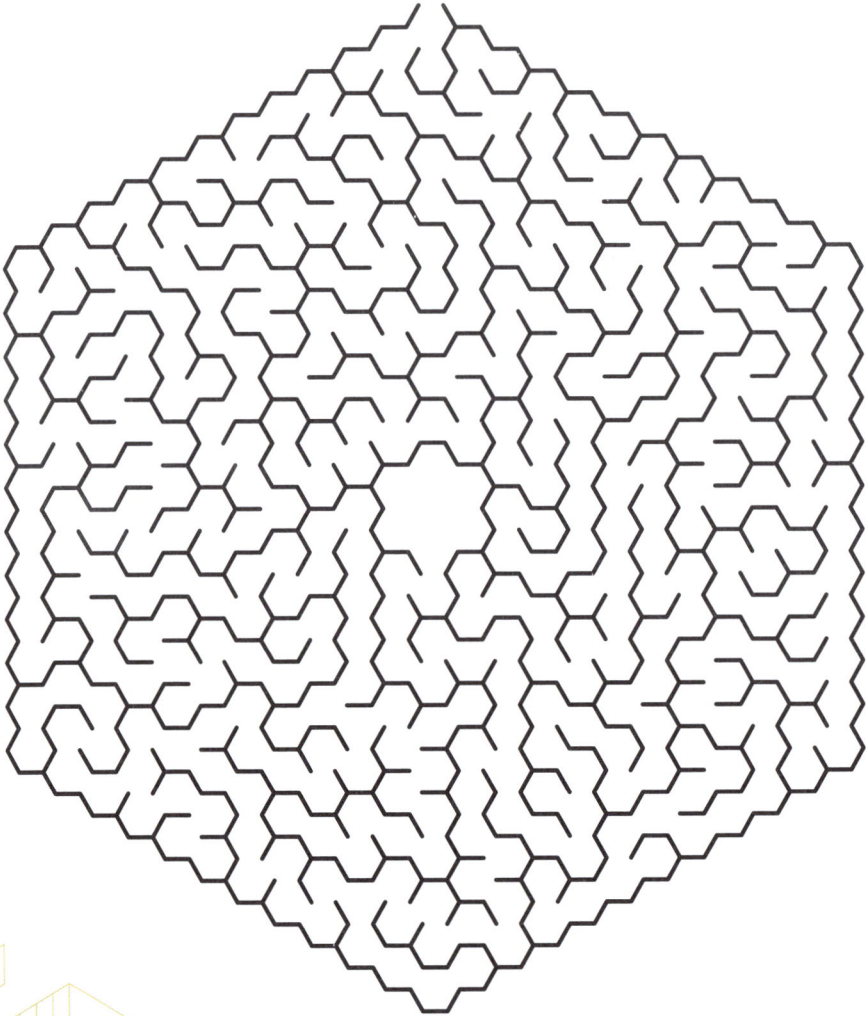

Maze 3

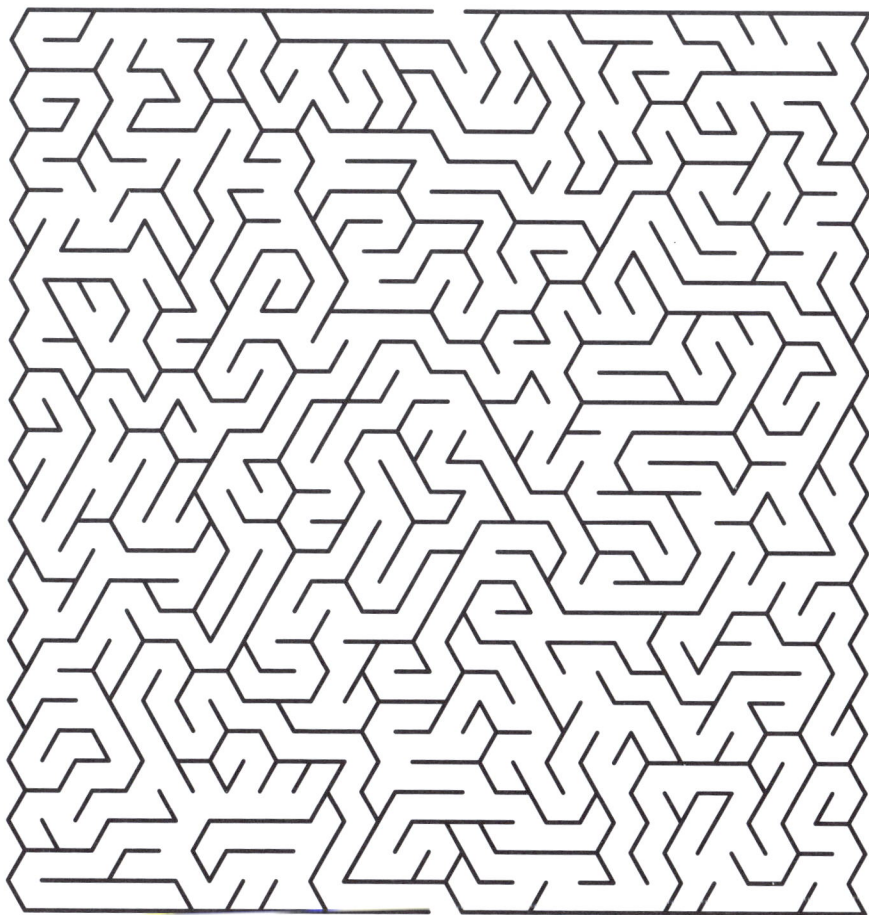
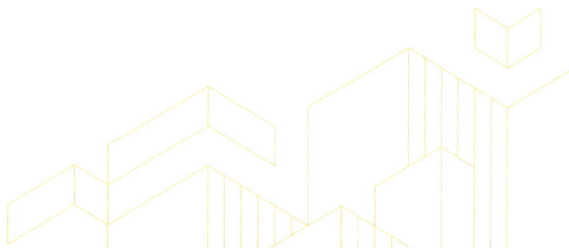

Sudoku 1

			8					9
	1	9			5	8	3	
	4	3		1				7
4			1	5				3
		2	7		4		1	
	8			9		6		
	7				6	3		
	3			7			8	
9		4	5					1

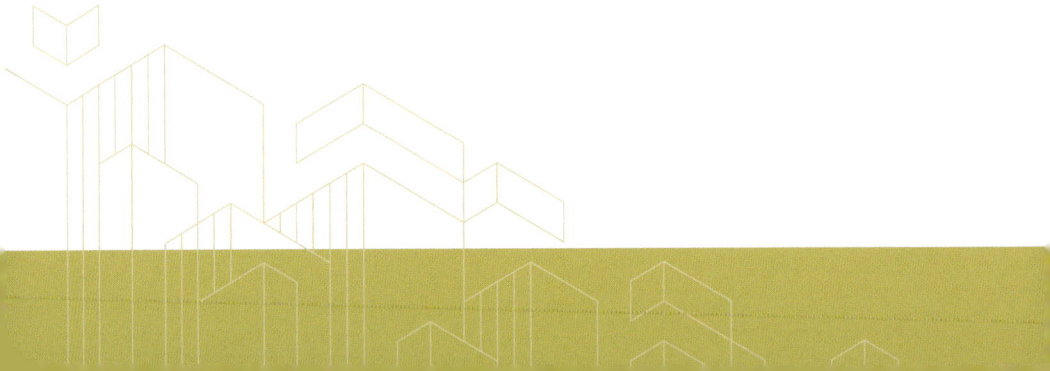

Sudoku 2

	6	3		2	7		8	
9				6		7		
			5	8	9		6	
1		7			8			
		9			5			
	8		9	3	1			7
					4		9	8
		2					5	
							7	6

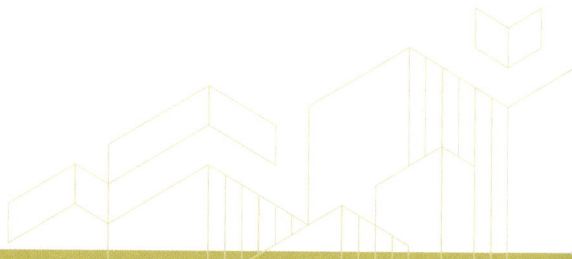

Sudoku 3

3					2	9		1
	6	8					3	2
9						8		5
		3	8	7		1		
		2				3	8	
		4	9		3	5	7	6
			2		1			
			6					
		9				6		

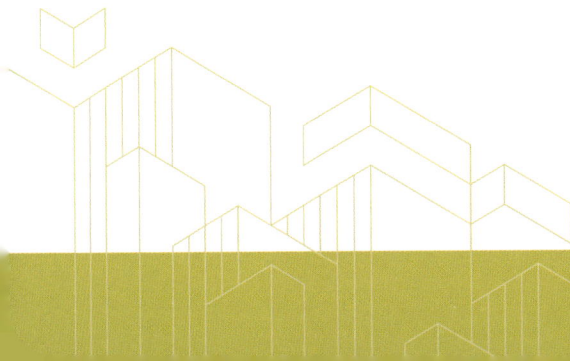

Word Search: Movie Genres

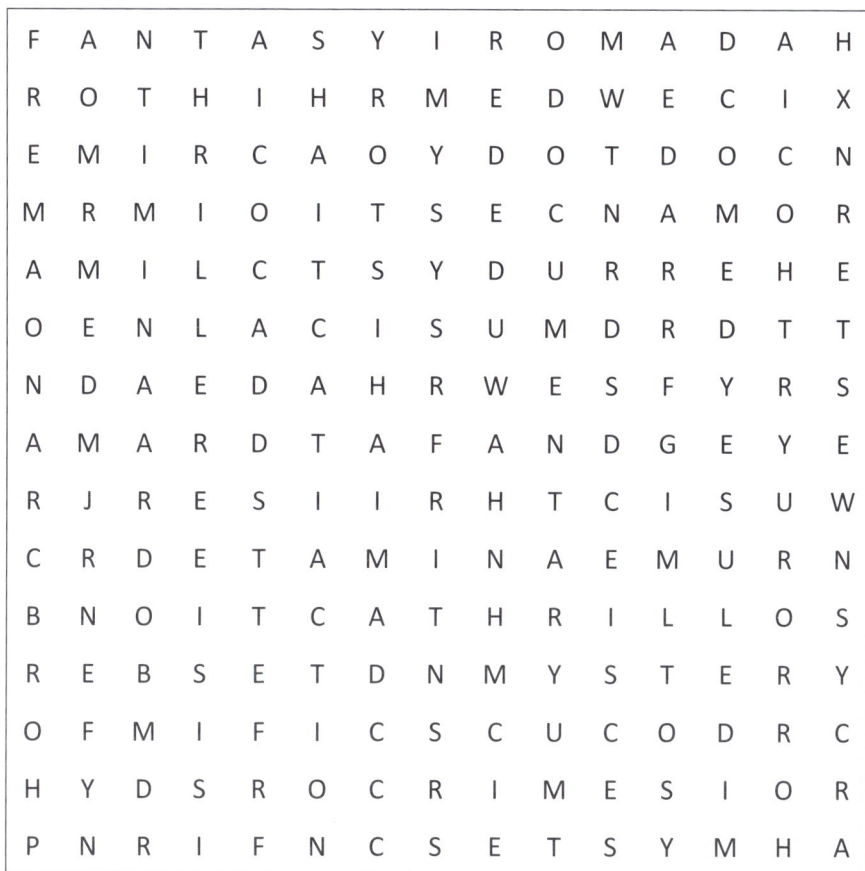

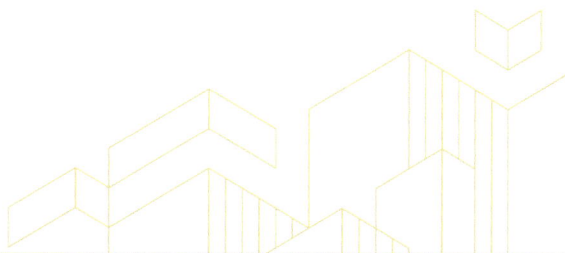

```
F  A  N  T  A  S  Y  I  R  O  M  A  D  A  H
R  O  T  H  I  H  R  M  E  D  W  E  C  I  X
E  M  I  R  C  A  O  Y  D  O  T  D  O  C  N
M  R  M  I  O  I  T  S  E  C  N  A  M  O  R
A  M  I  L  C  T  S  Y  D  U  R  R  E  H  E
O  E  N  L  A  C  I  S  U  M  D  R  D  T  T
N  D  A  E  D  A  H  R  W  E  S  F  Y  R  S
A  M  A  R  D  T  A  F  A  N  D  G  E  Y  E
R  J  R  E  S  I  I  R  H  T  C  I  S  U  W
C  R  D  E  T  A  M  I  N  A  E  M  U  R  N
B  N  O  I  T  C  A  T  H  R  I  L  L  O  S
R  E  B  S  E  T  D  N  M  Y  S  T  E  R  Y
O  F  M  I  F  I  C  S  C  U  C  O  D  R  C
H  Y  D  S  R  O  C  R  I  M  E  S  I  O  R
P  N  R  I  F  N  C  S  E  T  S  Y  M  H  A
```

Answers

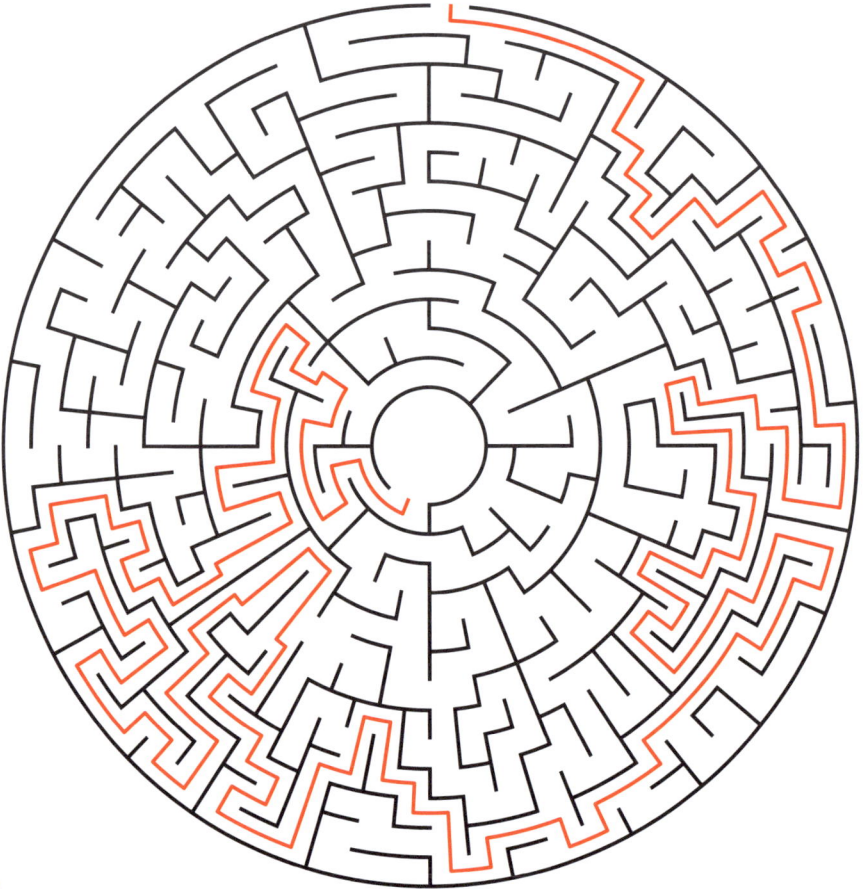

puzzle page 177

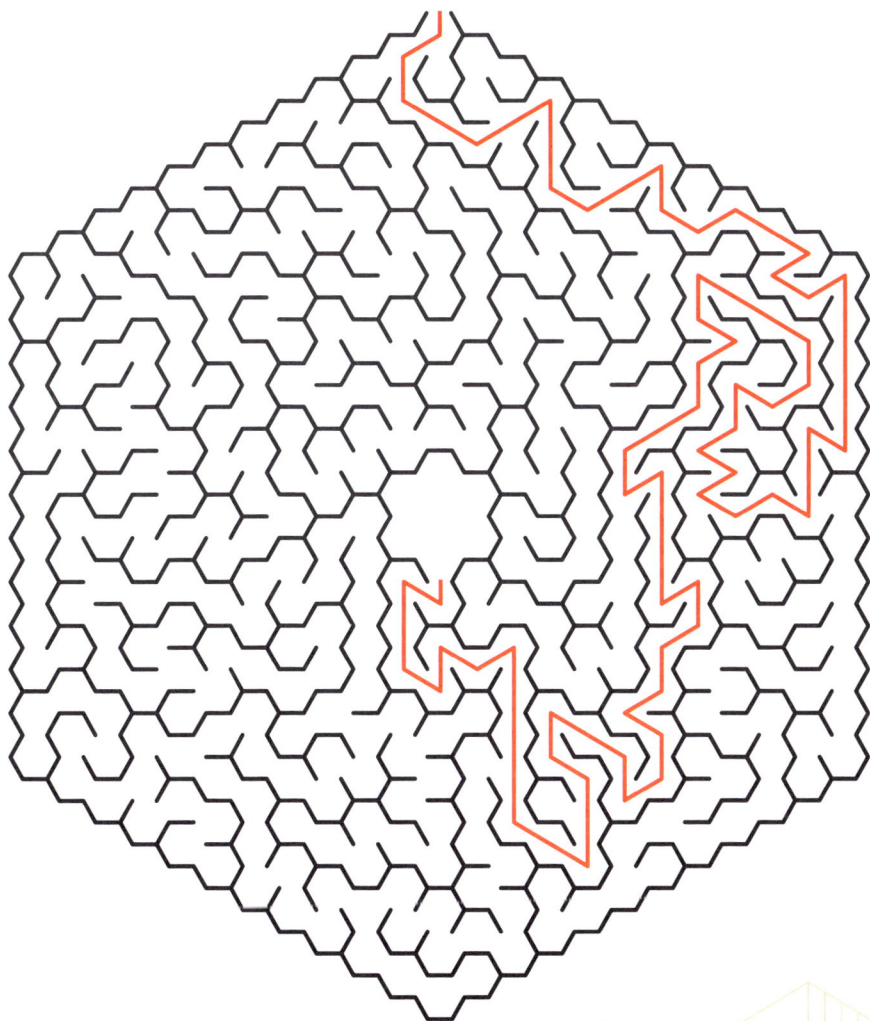

puzzle page 178

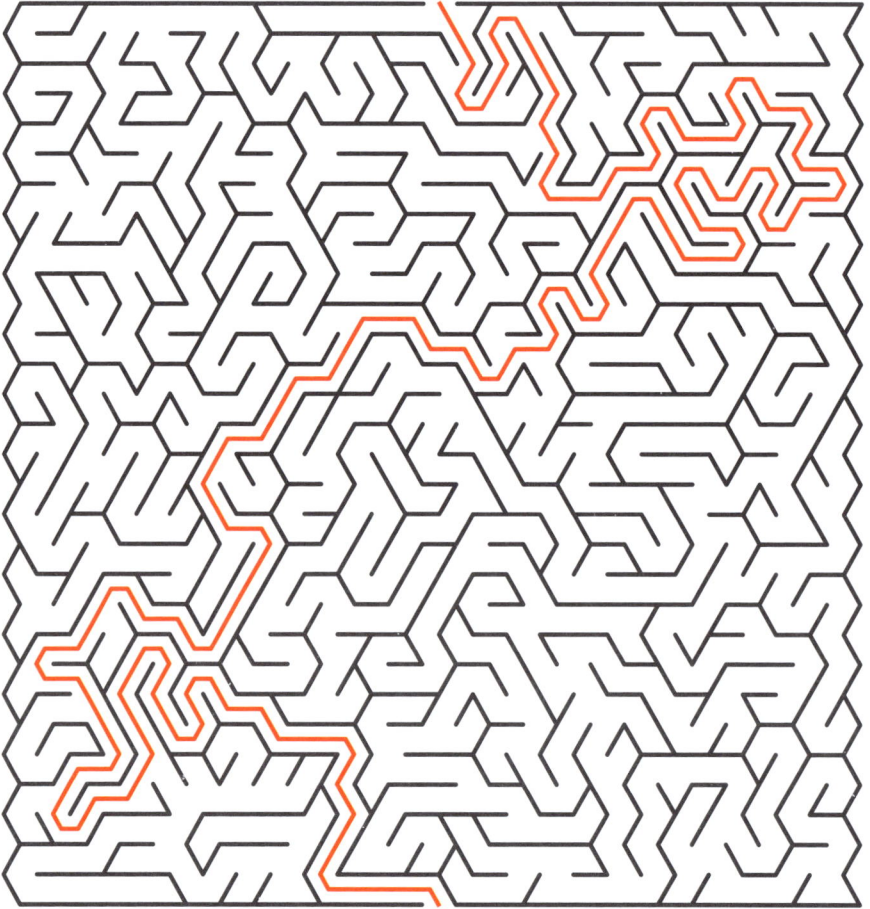

puzzle page 179

2	5	6	8	3	7	1	4	9
7	1	9	4	2	5	8	3	6
8	4	3	6	1	9	2	5	7
4	6	7	1	5	8	9	2	3
3	9	2	7	6	4	5	1	8
5	8	1	3	9	2	6	7	4
1	7	8	2	4	6	3	9	5
6	3	5	9	7	1	4	8	2
9	2	4	5	8	3	7	6	1

puzzle page 180

5	6	3	1	2	7	9	8	4
9	1	8	4	6	3	7	2	5
7	2	4	5	8	9	1	6	3
1	5	7	2	4	8	6	3	9
3	4	9	6	7	5	8	1	2
2	8	6	9	3	1	5	4	7
6	3	1	7	5	4	2	9	8
4	7	2	8	9	6	3	5	1
8	9	5	3	1	2	4	7	6

puzzle page 181

3	5	7	4	8	2	9	6	1
4	6	8	5	1	9	7	3	2
9	2	1	3	6	7	8	4	5
5	9	3	8	7	6	1	2	4
6	7	2	1	4	5	3	8	9
8	1	4	9	2	3	5	7	6
7	3	6	2	9	1	4	5	8
1	8	5	6	3	4	2	9	7
2	4	9	7	5	8	6	1	3

puzzle page 182

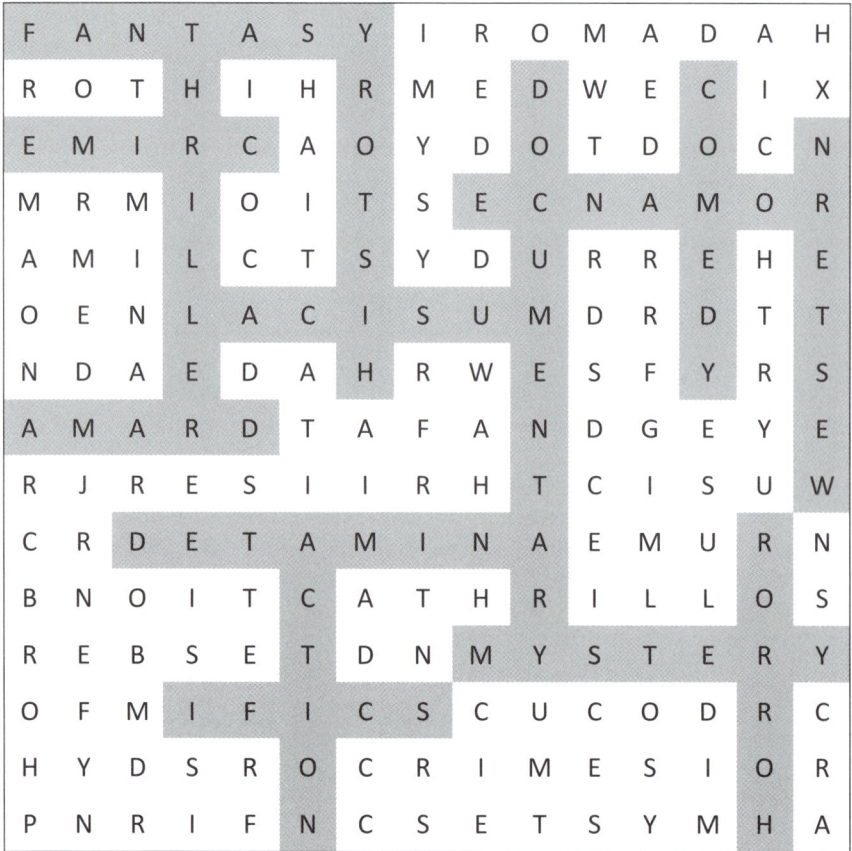

F	A	N	T	A	S	Y	I	R	O	M	A	D	A	H
R	O	T	H	I	H	R	M	E	D	W	E	C	I	X
E	M	I	R	C	A	O	Y	D	O	T	D	O	C	N
M	R	M	I	O	I	T	S	E	C	N	A	M	O	R
A	M	I	L	C	T	S	Y	D	U	R	R	E	H	E
O	E	N	L	A	C	I	S	U	M	D	R	D	T	T
N	D	A	E	D	A	H	R	W	E	S	F	Y	R	S
A	M	A	R	D	T	A	F	A	N	D	G	E	Y	E
R	J	R	E	S	I	I	R	H	T	C	I	S	U	W
C	R	D	E	T	A	M	I	N	A	E	M	U	R	N
B	N	O	I	T	C	A	T	H	R	I	L	L	O	S
R	E	B	S	E	T	D	N	M	Y	S	T	E	R	Y
O	F	M	I	F	I	C	S	C	U	C	O	D	R	C
H	Y	D	S	R	O	C	R	I	M	E	S	I	O	R
P	N	R	I	F	N	C	S	E	T	S	Y	M	H	A

Your Blueprint for a Longer, Healthier Life

You've reached the end of The Longevity Blueprint. Remember that longevity isn't about a single habit, supplement, or shortcut. It's the product of consistent, intentional choices that work together to strengthen your body, mind, and spirit.

Nutrition lays the foundation. The foods you choose fuel every cell, influence your hormones, and protect you from chronic disease. A diet rich in whole, nutrient-dense ingredients support energy, immunity, and long-term vitality.

Exercise builds on that foundation, keeping muscles strong, bones dense, and the cardiovascular system efficient. Movement is both a preventive measure and a celebration of what your body can do.

Sleep is the silent architect of longevity: repairing tissues, balancing hormones, and resetting the brain for optimal performance. Protecting your rest is as essential as your workouts or meals.

Mental stimulation ensures your brain stays agile and adaptable. By challenging yourself with new skills, games, and learning, you're not just preserving memory, you're expanding your capacity for joy, creativity, and problem-solving.

Mindfulness and meditation tie these elements together, training your attention, calming your nervous system, and helping you live with greater presence. Stress will always exist, but how you respond to it can mean the difference between burnout and balance.

Longevity isn't about adding more years to life. It's about adding more life to your years. The tools in this workbook are here for you to revisit, refine, and adapt as your journey evolves. Each small, consistent choice becomes part of your personal blueprint—a design for not just surviving, but thriving.

Your healthiest, longest life is built one mindful step at a time. The blueprint is in your hands—now it's up to you to live it.

Resources

Bregman, Peter. *The Bregman Method: A Proven Way to Banish Burnout, Sleep Deprivation, and Stress*. New York: Simon & Schuster, 2020.
A comprehensive guide to managing stress, improving mental clarity, and achieving peak productivity through lifestyle changes and practical techniques.

Cowan, Alex. *The Bulletproof Diet: Lose up to a Pound a Day, Reclaim Energy and Focus, Upgrade Your Life*. New York: Rodale Books, 2014.
This book discusses the Bulletproof Diet, a bio-hacking approach designed to optimize nutrition for mental and physical performance.

Doidge, Norman. *The Brain That Changes Itself: Stories of Personal Triumph from the Frontiers of Brain Science*. New York: Viking, 2007.
This groundbreaking book reveals how the brain is capable of rewiring itself, offering insights on how individuals can enhance cognitive function and overcome mental limitations.

Huberman, Andrew D. *The Huberman Lab Podcast*. Spotify, 2021–present.
A podcast that explores neuroscience, physiology, and bio-hacking practices with evidence-based recommendations for enhancing mental and physical health.

Hyman, Mark. The UltraMind Solution: *Fix Your Broken Brain by Healing Your Body First*. New York: Scribner, 2009.
This book links body health with mental clarity and offers practical advice on nutrition, lifestyle, and supplements to improve cognitive function.

Kelly, Dave Asprey. Game Changers: *What Leaders, Innovators, and Mavericks Do to Win at Life*. New York: Hay House, 2020.
Asprey, founder of Bulletproof, presents interviews with top performers about their own bio-hacking routines and strategies for achieving optimal brain and body health.

Ratey, John J. Spark: *The Revolutionary New Science of Exercise and the Brain*. New York: Little, Brown and Company, 2008.
Ratey explores the science behind how physical exercise boosts brain function, from increasing neuroplasticity to enhancing memory, focus, and overall cognitive health.

Wilkes, Ben. *The 4-Hour Body: An Uncommon Guide to Rapid Fat-Loss, Incredible Sex, and Becoming Superhuman*. New York: Crown Publishing Group, 2010.
Tim Ferriss's exploration into bio-hacking techniques focused on optimizing the body for fat loss, muscle gain, sleep, and overall well-being.